Your copy of *Managed Care Ethics:*
Essays on the Impact of Managed Care
on Traditional Medical Ethics
was made possible
by an unrestricted educational grant
from Zeneca Pharmaceuticals.

MANAGED CARE ETHICS

Essays on the Impact of Managed Care on Traditional Medical Ethics

JOHN LA PUMA, M.D.

A Hatherleigh CME book

HATHERLEIGH PRESS

New York

Hatherleigh Press
1114 First Avenue, Suite 500
New York, NY 10021
1-800-906-1234

Library of Congress Cataloging-in-Publication Data

LaPuma, John.
Managed care ethics: essays on the impact of managed care on traditional medical ethics/John LaPuma.
p. cm.—(A Hatherleigh CME book)
Includes bibliographical references and index.
ISBN 1-57826-012-4 (hardcover: alk. paper)
1. Managed care plans (Medical care)—moral and ethical aspects.
2. Medical ethics—Practice. I. Title. II. Series. III. Series:
A Hatherleigh CME book.
[DNLM: 1. Ethics, Medical—United States. 2. Managed Care Programs—United States. 3. Decision Making. 4. Ethics, Medical—United States.
5. Managed Care Programs—United States. 6. Decision Making.
W 50 L317m 1997]
R725.5.L3 1997
174'.2—dc21   97-41350
                                                              CIP

Printed in Canada

Designed by Dede Cummings Designs

10   9   8   7   6   5   4   3   2

ABOUT THE AUTHOR

J OHN LA PUMA practices general internal medicine in Chicago and first joined an Independent Practice Association in 1987. The first physician to enter a postgraduate fellowship in clinical ethics, he founded and directed the Lutheran General Center for Clinical Ethics and has testified before the United States Senate, the Brookings Institute and the Annenberg Foundation. He serves on The Robert Wood Johnson National Task Force on End of Life Care in Managed Care and has written a monthly ethics column for *Managed Care—A Guide for Physicians* since 1994. His work has been published by *The New England Journal of Medicine*, *The New York Times*, *The Encyclopedia Britannica* and *The Wall Street Journal*.

Dr. La Puma is also a professional chef. He works at Frontera Grill/Topolobampo in Chicago on Fridays with Chef Rick Bayless and leads the Cooking, Healthy Eating and Fitness (C.H.E.F.) Solution^SM Program at Alexian Brothers Medical Center in Elk Grove Village, Illinois. With David Schiedermayer, M.D., Dr. La Puma has also written *The McGraw-Hill Pocket Guide to Managed Care: Business, Practice, Law, Ethics* (Practice Management Information Corporation, Los Angeles, 1996) and *Ethics Consultation: A Practical Guide* (Jones and Bartlett, Boston, 1994).

Dr. La Puma can be reached at j-la-puma@uchicago.edu.

DEDICATION

For my father,
who taught me to do what was right
and my mother,
who helped me do it.

CONTENTS

ACKNOWLEDGMENTS

I have had many wonderful teachers and incurred several large debts of gratitude while completing this book. I am grateful to Tim Kelley and Tim Stezzi at *Managed Care—A Guide for Physicians* for their faith, vision and fairness, and their thoughtfulness from the very beginning of our partnership. I am also grateful to Andrew Flach of The Hatherleigh Company for his enthusiasm for a short, friendly guide to managed care ethics, and to Preston Williams for his inspirational belief in doing good in the face of adversity. I am also grateful to Mary Bennett, Diane Bishop Nobles, Drs. David Nash and David Schiedermayer for their knowledge and generosity, and to Pat Paulson, Kelley Clancy and Mary Doherty of Alexian Brothers Medical Center for their support.

Finally, Jeanne McMahon's love and kindness are very special gifts to me, and I am especially grateful for them.

MANAGED CARE ETHICS

*Essays on the Impact of Managed Care
on Traditional Medical Ethics*

INTRODUCTION

I believe that physicians can practice honorable, first-rate medicine in managed care. I also believe that they need a new set of ethics and communication and management skills to do it.

That is why I wrote this book: to help you organize your thinking about common ethical issues in managed care. Some issues are unique to capitation. Others are part of working with and for a managed care organization. Still others are part of every clinician-patient relationship. All can be pinpointed, placed squarely on the table and thought through.

Many of the chapters in this book have previously appeared as monthly ethics columns in the periodical *Managed Care—A Guide for Physicians*. I have adapted them for this format, which concludes with a Continuing Medical Education supplement worth nine Category 1 credits.

Managed care ethics is neither an oxymoron nor a euphemism for toeing the line. It is an explanation of how managed care can do good by doing more to uphold the values that matter most to patients, families and physicians.

Currently, managed care is a system that strives to provide the cheapest option available—not the most efficient or best quality or most cost-effective. But managed care should strive to be the

Gap, the Motorola, the Neiman-Marcus of health care systems, not the Dollar Store. Its service should be first rate, and its concern about costs should be invisible behind its love of quality. Its profits should provide access to care for those who are uninsured and underinsured.

The current moral vulnerability of managed care has created an opportunity for physicians to make better ethical decisions in and about managed care than they ever have. New, difficult conflicts of interest involving business, money and patient care will present themselves in the future. If physicians are skeptical, savvy and smart, they can help create a better future for managed care patients and for those who cannot yet afford managed care.

Patients trust managed care little, fear the loss of their jobs a lot and doubt that doctors would fight the managed care company on their behalf if push came to shove. But a physician is still a patient's best advocate, and *can* make a difference—by staying on the right side of the ethical road, now cratered with minimalist moral standards and money-back guarantees.

Most clinicians are deeply concerned about doing the right thing. Those who are well informed, who help patients take their health into their own hands, who recognize and document what a patient needs and why, who fight for what is right, and who organize with others to practice can make managed care into a system that works hard to prevent disease, promote health, and care for people when they are well and when they are ill. This future can be ours—it is up to us to take it back.

PART 1

1

The Rise
of Patient Autonomy

*Mrs. Clocker had lung cancer five and a half years ago and ran the Boston
Marathon last month. This month she is dying. She does not understand
how this could happen. She had the surgery, of course. She took all of the
chemo without a word. She ate only organic vegetables and grains and free-
range chicken. She went back to teaching English. She was "essentially
cured." She is 54.*

    *Now she is in the hospital, and someone else is here to take more
blood. She is told she must have a transfusion and take more chemo.
Why? How could this happen? Why do they keep taking blood? No
wonder she needs a transfusion! Why must she take more chemo? Why?
Where is my doctor, she thinks. "I want to see Dr. Beale," she tells the
nurse. "Nothing until then. Nothing."*

THE MEANING of "autonomy" has changed dramati-
cally in medicine over the past 50 years. It has gone from
meaning that it is wrong to experiment on people without their consent to meaning that patients have the moral right to
request physician assistance in suicide.

    But autonomy is not a free ride. Being free from interfer-
ence from others also implies some duties—not harming other

people, not infringing on their freedom, not hogging society's resources.

Is more autonomy good or bad for patients in managed care?
What do more patient preferences now mean for the availability of
care later? Has patient autonomy been replaced by the pressure of
time and financial incentives? Could capitation mean more choice
for more people?

How has autonomy changed in recent years?

Autonomy has become the most important ethical principle in
modern medicine—more than beneficence, integrity, justice, or
respect for persons. But this is a very recent change.

Before the Nuremberg trials midcentury, a physician's beneficent effort to do good was good enough for first place in medical
ethics. Patient autonomy was tied for second place with justice,
from which it was inseparable. The preferences and potential
choices of any one patient were limited by the number of medications the physician had to offer and how many house calls he or
she still had to make. Though they could be severed, autonomy
and justice travelled together.

And that has been the change in autonomy in managed care.
Freed from its link to justice, autonomy is flying high. It is choice,
control, customer-oriented and full of freedom for one's self and
one's family. The civil rights movements of the '60s and '70s, the
gay rights and disability rights movements of the '80s and the se-
nior rights movement of the '90s predicted that patient preferences would reign supreme.

As patients made themselves heard—for choices of better pain
relief, for choices near the end of life, for choices of no-repeat
Cesarean section and breast-sparing cancer surgery—physician autonomy has dwindled. A lot.

Too many physicians lost respect for true patient autonomy,
making science and certainty their mantra, and health care costs
zoomed. Employee health benefits disappeared, and so did the
flexibility to make medical decisions purely medical. Sadly, too
many physicians will also cede their clinical authority to politicians

and their basic livelihood to business people, some of whom are bandits. And bandits have already stolen issues about which physicians should be leaders.

Relief of pain and suffering near the end of life is one such issue. Every physician can prevent the invasion of last-moment medical technology that serves only to delay a patient's death. Every physician can recognize that a devastating stroke, not a decision to honor a family's request to discontinue a mechanical ventilator, is the cause of that patient's death. These are issues that physicians already understand and act on, and should champion for patients.

Another such issue, and indeed a controversial one, is euthanasia. It is paradoxical that there is a touted "right to die" when the only absolute right to medical treatment is in federal prisons. What medical justification could there be for killing a patient? What indication or contraindication? Too easily in medicine can a wish to respect a patient's wishes become a wish to ease a family's suffering when the patient's wishes are unknown and unknowable. That shaded, distorted judgment has crept up on physicians in the Netherlands and Australia. Are U.S. physicians so different?

American physicians are not different. **They should become experts in relieving pain and suffering, not at assisting suicide and committing euthanasia. To promote genuine patient autonomy, *shared decision-making*—not unilateral judgments—should become the rule.**

Prior to managed care, there was only patient compliance: a one-way directive. The difference between compliance and adherence, which is what there is now, is the difference between agreement and obligation. Adherence is how many physicians now think of what they and their patients attempt to create, and at the center of that accommodation is patient accountability.

Accountability and autonomy should go hand in hand in managed care, just like choices and consequences. Managed care is all about self-reliance, self-motivation and enlightened self-interest. It has autonomy, adherence and accountability written all over it. And so do the solutions to the most common causes of death and disability. Smoking, obesity, sedentariness, alcohol abuse and drug use are problems of epidemic proportion that patients can and should decide to overcome.

Yet deciding is not enough, and so disease management and patient education programs can demonstrate that autonomy carries accountability with it. Clinicians can offer patients effective tools for beating lifestyle habits that are currently beating them. It will be up to patients to use these tools and up to creative managed care to offer them incentives for so doing.

Some physicians are not permitted to use their most powerful tool—talk. They have powerful incentives not to use it: fear of termination if the truth slips out about what is covered, what is available and what is not. Yet "gag rules" are less of a problem than "anti-disparagement clauses," which seek to silence physicians before they speak. Some physicians are unable to cut these clauses from contracts, and see no choice but to sign. Yet autonomy means little without truth-telling.

Confidentiality means little without truth-telling too, and it is a decrepit concept in medical care. The 72 people who see a physician's diagnosis of depression before it gets to the mental health triage worker can be counted. Not so with the dozens who can wander up to a permanently logged-on terminal, day or night. Or the hundreds of associates who share the same log-in number to a health system. Or the curious handful who want to know about that recently admitted rock star's review of systems.

The real issue about confidentiality in managed care is contained in one phrase: employer database. The data mining and warehousing industry looks at lists of names, addresses and diagnoses like so much coal: dump them in bins and sell them by the truckload. Compressed onto tapes and drives, they shine like the diamonds they are. Discriminated against for a promotion? Tested recently for genetic linkages to Alzheimer's? Can't get insurance? See the connection?

Financial incentives to gather, buy and sell personal information do not conflict with federal privacy standards, because there are none. There are none! Billing services, health plans and pharmaceutical houses already can use new information systems to profiteer while making a mockery of patient privacy.

There can be no privacy or therapeutic bond without trust, and patients still want to trust. So do physicians. There are often moments in which a patient leans close or averts his eyes and says, "This is just between us, right?" Those moments are times in which putting down the pen lets the physician listen just a little better and decide with the patient what goes in the record and what doesn't.

Because an individual physician often makes this intimate effort with a patient who needs it, and because professionalism and self-esteem are so important, the idea of disclosing to a patient how and how much the physician is paid seems irrelevant. Why do patients need to know about the physician's interest in financial and job security? What attorney or university professor or restauranteur tells his or her clients or students or customers about incentives to spend more time or do less teaching or close early?

For physicians, capitation, which is payment per member per time, represents a huge ethical dilemma and poisons discussions of patient preference because physicians seem to have so little choice themselves about how to care for patients. Capitation seems to narrow choices to those available by contract, not by covenant. Some financial incentives seem too much for any physician to bear: very small risk pools, very large sums withheld, very few colleagues with whom to share risk. No physicians should take them or be subject to them, because all are only human.

If physicians remain patient advocates, they cannot avoid difficult financial decisions and conflicts of interest. But physicians are the best advocates that patients have—and the only ones who care primarily about patient well-being. What is autonomy, physicians reason, if it isn't choice of physician?

To many patients, autonomy is not choice of physician: it is choice of health plan. This is a step backward, for it should not be either/or, but both. Point of service plans, preferred provider organizations and open panel HMOs can solve some problems of autonomy and should be encouraged: There is evidence that enrollment in them is on the way up. Yet employers in the 1980s spoke loud and clear about their outrageous costs, and demanded fewer treatments with fewer complications from their health plans. The tradeoff for patients: loss of choice of physician.

For patients to make autonomous choices, they must know how their insurance works. Many do, and choose: "Yes" to less paperwork and lower co-payments; "No" to long waits and less personalness. Patients go to or come from oncologists and receive visits from home health personnel their primary physician does not know, has not met and cannot vouch for, even near the end of life.

Doing less near the end of life is particularly problematic in capitated managed care. On the one hand, survey after survey shows that most patients value quality of life as much as or more than survival. On the other hand, managed care is not trusted to deliver quality end-of-life care, because of the cold, financial fear that plans may suddenly "honor" a patient's preferences for withdrawing treatment that are not that patient's preferences at all.

An easy way to honor patient autonomy and to save money would appear to be to honor advance directives. Living wills are advance directives, yet chances are three out of four that if a hospitalized patient has one, clinicians will know nothing about it. Few advance directives make it to the medical record, and once there, few directives are clear enough for clinicians to use.

Advance directives may or may not save money and are often useless in the hospital and nursing home except as a flag for the need for advance care planning. Especially with an advance directive in hand, the doctor must still review with the patient his or her reasons, preferences and choices. Planning is a clinical responsibility, not a marketing or accounting one. Clinicians should take this responsibility because it promotes patient choice, offers hope and opens a door to participation when disease processes may be beyond their control. It also protects against lawsuits.

Giving hope even when there seems to be no reason for hope and remaining at the patient's side when everyone else has left can give profound joy to others. Doing the right thing at the right time for the right reason—taking time with a patient and family to make good choices in light of what matters most to them—forms the enduring backbone of what physicians do. This is as true in managed care as it is in any other system.

Autonomy in managed care: the road ahead

That afternoon, Dr. Beale had messages from the nurse, utilization management, the HMO medical director, Mrs. Clocker's husband, and two of her three daughters. He went back to the hospital at 8 p.m., walked in the room and looked at gaunt, tough Mrs. Clocker staring at him.

"This has been a hard day for you, hasn't it?" Dr. Beale said.

Mrs. Clocker's folded arms and tight jaw eased a little. If he could see what she could see! Her daughters without their mother, her students without their present participles, her running shoes without her. Fear and disappointment overcame her. Tears welled up.

"I would be surprised if someone with a cancer in the lung wasn't frightened," Dr. Beale said, sitting down. "We have some choices to make."

Autonomy has had a meteoric rise, and it's still on the way up. Much of this rise is good—**the more patients know about the care they and their employer have purchased, the better decisions they can make.** But unbounded autonomy is not good—resources are still limited, and individuals and their families do not live in a vacuum. They cannot lunch every day at a community buffet of endless individual portions.

The concept of shared responsibility for medical health and financial well-being challenges the rugged individualism and immediate gratification of turn-of-the-century America. We want a Range Rover for city streets and a living will in case we fall ill and Fat-Free Pringles for any time at all.

But can't we have Pringles and eat them too? Indeed we can. And we have. That's the problem. We haven't accepted the consequences of our choices. But they are coming. Fast.

What can clinicians do to promote patients' autonomy and, at the same time, help them think of themselves as members of a community?

1. Honor autonomy when it is about personal choices. Make sure the information patients have is not misinformation gleaned from television spots and department store displays. Learn from patients' experiments with alternative treatments, and share information with colleagues about better practices. Document patients' desires to choose their own course.

2. Solicit patient preference by asking for patients' opinions, understandings, interpretations and own words. Say "What do you think it is?" or "Tell me more about that" or "Go on" or "What else?" or "What do you think about taking this new medicine?" Don't wait for patients to ask. Ask them. These questions emphasize physicians' interest in patients' ideas.

3. Utilize a separate, advance planning office visit for discussion of palliative care. Ideally, it should be conducted with the patient and the proxy decision-maker in a 30-minute visit. The complexity, intensity, duration and personal nature of the issues should be documented clearly.

4. Know that physician-assisted suicide (PAS) can vary from state to state, but for now, it is illegal in every state except Oregon; that withdrawing or withholding life-sustaining treatment is legally different than PAS; and that physicians who administer adequate pain relief and seek to alleviate intractable pain, even if a patient dies as a result.

5. Share the responsibility for doing more with less. Try, "We have a few minutes to discuss your most important problem today." If a second or third unrelated problem is raised, try, "This new problem is important, and I want to give it all the time you think it needs. Can it wait until next time?"

2

The Dawning of the Age of Accountability

A U T O N O M Y has transformed medical ethics in just half a century. Gone is beneficence-based medical ethics in which the doctor knows and acts for the patient's good, and patients do their best to get better. Earlier in this century, our country had more of a sense of community, togetherness and scarcity. Not everyone could have everything, and we knew it.

In the place of do-good medical ethics has come me-first medical ethics. Many patients know more about their conditions, as they should, but worry more too. Some worry about the little things—a headache could be a brain tumor—but miss the big picture: Their obesity exacerbates their hypertension. As often as not, patients worry just about themselves, without acknowledging their community or its limits.

For the 21st century, the 20th-century concept of patient autonomy will prove inadequate. The single doctor-single patient relationship cannot provide enough care for all who need it.

One-quarter of New York City residents under 65 have no insurance; most have full-time jobs. Those fortunate enough to have insurance must be willing to share, because autonomy without justice is just selfish. We cannot afford to care just about ourselves and our families anymore.

The reality is that we have tough choices and finite resources. Discussions of managed care ethics must now include the principles of accountability and fairness to others. **Patients should be accountable for managing and preventing diseases that are largely within their control.** Patients who either choose to ignore physician advice about their medication and life styles, or will not learn the necessary skills or deny the inevitable consequences of diabetes and hypertension are acting autonomously *at the expense of others, as well as themselves.*

Likewise, physicians should be accountable for sound advice and good service to their patients. Physicians should create medical forums inside their offices for helping patients prevent illness and complications in organized, prevention-oriented programs. Managed care physicians who educate their patients will be busier than ever.

Patient commitment

Why should patients be more accountable for managing their own diseases? Here are some financial reasons.

If you're a smoker, let's say you'll save $700 cash annually if you stop smoking and test negative for plasma nicotine. If you're a diabetic, let's say you'll save $800 annually if your random glycohemoglobin is less than 8 percent. Would you consider changing your behavior and planning to take control of your care?

Here are popular reasons some people do consider changing. The Marcus Welby doctor-dependent patient paradigm changed decades ago. People are no longer dependent on physicians for medical information. Talk radio and television started this revolution. The Internet and vitamin displays at drugstores may likely finish it. There isn't an American adult who doesn't know that tobacco and lung disease are related.

Take dinner, for example. Supersizing is killing us. When I was growing up, dinner plates were nine inches; today, they're 13 inches, sometimes more. Portions more than fill our extra large plates. More is better, it seems. More is not cheaper, however, as the true price of a 55-cent Big Mac depends upon the CPT code for angioplasty.

Obesity? Thirty-three percent and climbing. Hyperlipidemia? Rampant. Diabetes? Epidemic.

Physician commitment

Why should physicians be more accountable for preventing disease?

Here are some financial reasons.

If you're capitated for 100,000 lives, you want the water to be pure and food safety to be high. You want sexually transmitted diseases and resistant organisms reported. You want Joe Camel six feet under and cigarettes out of sports arenas. You want 2-percent milk to be called what it is, which is 38 percent of calories from fat.

You want mandatory seatbelt and helmet laws. You want people to change some lifestyle habits and mean it. You don't want to pay for other people's carelessness out of your patients' money.

You want your patients to schedule regular office visits, attend smoking cessation courses, and investigate yoga and mind-body techniques to manage stress and hypertension. Making it easy for patients to prevent disease and to invest in their own health is good service, good medicine and worth compensating explicitly.

Two principles in partnership

Accountability should partner with autonomy as the most important principle in managed care ethics. Insisting that patients take proactive, positive steps to change what and how they eat, when and where and how often they exercise, whether they smoke and how much they drink can work for physicians who feel their time is wasted unless the patient gets serious about his or her disease.

Is accountability a viable partner for autonomy in this age of get-ahead, me-first, you-second, faster, quicker, better?

Accountability and managed care ethics are about control and choice—our favorite American values. Self-reliance and enlightened self-interest for both patients and physicians have "self" written all over them.

Yet invoking "accountability" is not a panacea. It will not get the government out of the examining room, or reossify osteoporotic hips. No physician wants to abandon patients unable or unwilling to help themselves. No patient wants to have diabetes or hypertension or heart disease.

But accountability is not about abandonment or blaming the victim. It is about resource allocation and fairness. Too many people covered by managed care have medical problems that they can address but do not. Too many people outside of managed care want in, but cannot get in. Emphasizing wellness could make more room.

What to do?

- Tell patients that control of their health is in their own hands. Offer them educational help.
- When you make a treatment contract with a patient, make sure the "deal" isn't personal, so you do not suffer if the patient fails.
- Notice the advertising in sports arenas and the FDA labels on animal food products—think of their negative impact on the capitated payments you may be receiving.
- Ask parents to model changes for their children, who learn primarily by their parents' example.
- Use gentle persistence when patients continue to smoke or refuse to exercise.
- Don't complain to or get angry at patients when they fail. It doesn't work.
- Relinquish the responsibility for healthful living to patients. Congratulate them when they accept it.

For Further Reading:

1. Darragh M, McCarrick PM. Scope Note 31: Managed health care: new ethical issues for all. Kennedy Institute of Ethics Journal 1996; 6(2):1–12.

2. Friedman E. Making choices: coming home to roost. Health-care Forum Journal 1997 January/February; 11–13.
3. Sennett C. Establishing accountability in managed health care. in Seltzer J, Nash DB. Models for Measuring Quality in Managed Care. Faulkner & Gray, New York, 1997, pp 36–54.

3

Accountability in Managed Care: What Should We Expect from Patients?

PERSONAL RESPONSIBILITY is the cornerstone of morality, and the building of every temple of modern bioethics has begun with that first stone. Similarly, disease prevention and health promotion are the foundations of managed care, and those concepts depend on people taking responsibility for their own health. In the 1990s, this means special attention to common, expensive, too often lethal and often preventable conditions—like tobacco dependence and obesity.

Writing in the Journal of the American Medical Association three years ago, Drs. McGinnis and Foege showed that smoking— not coronary disease or neoplasms—caused death in 33 percent of the cases they reviewed, more than any other factor. High-fat/low-carbohydrate-and-fiber diets and sedentary activity levels were second at 19 percent. Alcohol and drug abuse, firearms, motor vehicle accidents and sexual behavior were not far behind.

Many observers hope that significant behavioral change has begun. Many managed care organizations hope to increase efficiency with disease and demand management programs. Employers hope the popularity of wellness programs will result in lower costs. Physicians hope for a preventive intervention for sedentary fast food addicts that is as effective as first-dollar coronary artery bypass graft coverage.

Hope is important, but it is not always enough to pull patients through. How important to managed care ethics is personal responsibility? Should patients be held accountable for "risky behavior"? Or is this violating civil liberties or patients' rights to choose, or "blaming the victim"? After all, patients are sick people, and may have illnesses for which genes, heredity, environment, family, or fate is actually responsible.

The arguments for accountability

Here are three compelling reasons that support accountability: education, independence and equality.

With multimedia, from compact disc-containing books to interactive videos, from faxback technology and popular television to the Internet, the single most important source of a patient's information about his or her care has changed from medicine to the media.

Patients are less dependent upon physicians for knowledge and have become more autonomous decision-makers over the past 50 years. Yet their responsibility in the doctor-patient relationship has not increased proportionately.

Sociologist Talcott Parsons described the patient's "sick role" in the late 1940s—dependent, fearful, trusting in science. The patient's physician was learned, without conflict and generally always available to direct the patient's care. The patient did his or her best to get better. Care was inexpensive by today's standards, and bartering was usually still possible in a pinch.

By contrast, many of today's patients dislike the idea of orders from an authority and are accustomed to more egalitarian relationships with their health care providers. Patients are well aware of physicians' divided loyalties, too-limited schedules and near top-of-the-heap incomes. Often reasonably well when they negotiate for and purchase health care, patients and employers try to make hard-headed decisions about what they can afford, in part because care is so expensive and not the only thing of value.

There are other reasons for greater accountability. First is population-based health: Resources saved by one individual can be used
to benefit another in the population. Second is better communication: Ungagging physicians to discuss cost issues related to lifestyle
changes would help both doctors and patients to discuss patient values. Third is adequate access: Managed care patients no longer need
physicians to provide access, as the managed care organization provides that. Fourth is demonstrated cost-effectiveness and patient satisfaction, from self-help books to leading corporate fitness programs.

The arguments against accountability

**Here are three more reasons against accountability: dis-
crimination, privacy and uncertainty.**

Picking on alcohol and drug users and smokers can be viewed
as arbitrary and discriminatory. What about chronic skiers who
break a leg one year and return to Vail the next? Or motorcyclists
who ride with only tresses covering their naked heads across
Montana's speed-limitless beauty? Or balloonists who then try
hang-gliding or bungee-jumping? Why should one group be held
accountable for their injuries and potential injuries, and another be
held up as just adventurous?

Abusing alcohol and drugs, overeating, underexercising and
skiing are not medical behaviors. They are, in most cases, probably unrelated to taking medication or showing up for office visits.
Instead, they represent important value choices that people in this
country should be free to make. To control these activities with
rules or incentives would be parental and paternalistic. Physicians
are not charged with being enforcers of social policy, but instead
are compassionate advocates who put a particular patient, in the
office now, before personal or societal interest.

Scientific information about diet in particular seems to change
every month. The USDA creates and then retracts and then re-
issues a dietary Pyramid. It still lumps meat with beans and animal
fat with vegetable fat, and leaves out cooking methods and exercise. The new fat substitute, Olestra, may re-invent potato chips
even as it sucks folate and fluids from your system, not to mention

mouth-feel from your palate. And now there's leptin, which drains body weight from mice, and should be ready for FDA approval within 10 years. So why add 30 grams of fiber to your diet when the recommendation to do so could change any moment, and you may be able to take a fat pill?

There are other reasons here, too. First, patients are not really autonomous, even if they are better educated. More information can't always overcome genetics, luck and culture. Second, lifestyle behaviors are notoriously stubborn: Only one of 20 obese people who lose 20 pounds keeps it off for five years. Third, too many managed care organizations are more interested in short-term paybacks than long-term investments. And because patients change plans so often, any given managed care organization may be out of business and into Brazil by the time a comprehensive fitness program pays off.

So who is right?

Whichever side of the argument you find stronger, the issue of patient accountability is here to stay. **The real question is one of reins or fences—incentives or rules—and who constructs them, and why.** Physicians will seek new ways to align patient incentives with their own. In that way, perhaps, choice and information can reduce not only health care costs but also patient vulnerability.

For Further Reading:

1. DiMatteo MR, Sherbourne CD, Hays RD, et al. Physicians' characteristics influence patients' adherence to medical treatment: results from the Medical Outcomes Study. Health Psychology 1993; 12:93–102.
2. Houston Miller NH, Hill M, Kottke T, Ockene IS. The multilevel compliance challenge: recommendations for a call to action; a statement for health care professionals. Circulation 1997; 95:1085–1090.
3. Morreim EH. Lifestyles of the risky and infamous: from managed care to managed lives. Hastings Center Report 1995; 25(6):5–12.

4

When It's Hard to Be Sure
of the Patient's Own Goals

*Arlene Cass is a 43-year-old mother of two with a 10-year history of mul-
tiple sclerosis, admitted with aspiration pneumonia by her family physician. She and her family belong to a managed care organization. After
three days of hospital treatment, she was well enough to converse, and she
refused antibiotics and tube feeding.*

*Mrs. Cass said she did not wish to die. She was afraid of swallowing
and choking on her food, of losing control. "I like my mind," she said,
adding that she had had a full academic scholarship through college. "I
can't read now, with my vision gone, and I want to see my son graduate
college." She said she didn't want to end up like her uncle, who had had
severe Alzheimer's disease and had become unable to make decisions.*

*"Can I discharge her off antibiotics?" the family physician asked.
"On managed care rounds, utilization review pressured me to send her
out." That's when the hospital ethics consultant was called in.*

*On physical exam, the patient was an alert, bright-eyed woman with
severe skeletal deformities and diffuse muscle atrophy. She was unable to
move her extremities except her right arm. She had a five-centimeter stage
III sacral pressure sore. Her speech was slow and languorous, her affect sad,
her mood unhappy but her recent memory good.*

*The ethics consultant met with the patient's husband and two young
adult children. The husband said his wife was depressed and intellectually
frustrated. He wanted his wife to be given the feeding tube, believing that*

she was slightly confused and didn't know her own mind. But she denied that, telling the consultant, "I trust no one."

Under pressure from utilization management, the family physician had scheduled the patient for discharge the next day. The ethics consultant advised against this until the patient had more time to negotiate. Although it cost the managed care organization more money to continue the hospitalization, the consultant believed that her goals and objectives had not yet been heard.

During the patient's additional hospital stay, her attitudes and those of her doctors became more flexible. She said she would accept antibiotics and a feeding tube as long as she was mentally alert. With a new understanding of her priorities, the physicians soon stopped trying to press the feeding tube on her. In the end, she left the hospital without the feeding tube but with oral antibiotics.

T H E   C A S E of Arlene Cass shows the importance of clarifying the patient's own goals. Her values were not incorporated into the decision-making until she had improved enough to respond meaningfully to questions asked. Without her own choices on record, she might have been discharged too sick, too soon—perhaps to return to the hospital shortly. Other ethical issues raised by the case of Arlene Cass include:

- Patient autonomy, including how to elicit patients' choices, when to consider a family member's view of decision-making capacity, and what to do if the patient's choices conflict with fairness to other managed care enrollees;
- Financial incentives to limit care, how to confront them, when to share them with the patient and how to appeal them if they're unfair; and
- Treatment goals, their rationale and determining when hospitalization is consistent with them.

Managed care plans may ask physicians to limit the care some patients receive because of that care's cost. Patients like Arlene Cass may be among the first subjects of such requests, because their decision-making capacity is easily compromised by an infection or other minor medical problem.

Incentives to undertreat

The change from managing one patient to managing many, and from caring for the sickest first to caring for all equally, is unnatural for many physicians. This new approach may be distorted by some plans. In the worst cases, pure immediate cost containment drives a patient's early discharge, instead of a far-sighted, detailed view of the patient's goals and personal circumstances.

To resolve conflicts, managed care turns to standards: practice guidelines, outcomes research and quality assurance. Standards in ethics start with good clinical data and personal information—e.g., the patient's health care values and choices, and reasons for those choices. **Many believe that practice guidelines and physician accreditation standards, including some in ethics, will soon have economic teeth.**

Regardless of standards, most patients still expect doctors to be individual patient advocates first, usually without regard to the needs of other managed care members. They expect doctors to appeal economic constraints on their care to the medical director, the board of directors—even to Oprah Winfrey if need be.

When are such extreme steps warranted? **When appeals through traditional medical and administrative structures fail and the patient's medical interests are threatened, physicians can and should use the tradition of advocacy to our patients' advantage.** In the case of Arlene Cass, clarifying the patient's goals and negotiating with utilization management did the trick. We could save going to Oprah for another day.

For Further Reading:

1. Morreim EH. The ethics of incentives in managed care. Trends in Health Care, Law, and Ethics 1995; 10(1/2):56–62.
2. Rodwin MA. Conflicts in managed care. New England Journal of Medicine 1995; 332:602–606.
3. Rosenbaum S, Serrano R, Magar M, Stern G. Civil rights in a changing health system. Health Affairs 1997; 16(1):90–105.

5

Why Ethics Defines Quality—And Goals Define Ethics

IN THE OFFICE, clinic and hospital, practice guidelines play a larger role than ever. Are guidelines high-quality educational tools, or are they prescribed recipes, designed for idealized patients with the goal of saving the managed care plan money? Is using guidelines ethical?

Whether guidelines are educational or financial or helpful depends on what they say and how they are used, but that is not the case with ethics. Ethics is not fundamentally different in managed care than in any other financing or delivery system. It is still a flexible tool for decision-making that practitioners can use if they know how, and it is still anchored by the doctor-patient relationship. Identifying and resolving ethical issues is still part of the quality of care.

Three things about ethics, however, are different. **In managed care, patients are more likely to be undertreated than overtreated, because financial incentives now exist to undertreat.** The underlying framework in managed care is improving the health of a population, instead of focusing on an individual patient. And the desired settings for treatment are now the office and the home. They're cheaper than the hospital, and they are where more and more ethical issues are being transferred.

These three differences—financial incentives to limit treatment, population-based practice and shift in location of care—suggest several reasons why practice guidelines have gained such importance among managed care plans. Physicians themselves have seen the suffering of their patients, and often said "yes" when trying to relieve it. Physicians have said "yes" to more testing and another treatment, "yes" to more visits and regular re-assessments. This practice style does not fit most practice guidelines, however, and it is one reason that guidelines have gained prominence in managed care plans.

Doctors' traditional approach

For years, we physicians ordered "extra" tests and treatments to meet our own need (and sometimes the patient's request) for certainty. We ordered more with the hope of getting sued less, and in accordance with the principle of patient autonomy. Dotting every investigational "i" and crossing every therapeutic "t" has, until recently, been considered thoughtful, careful medical practice.

Similarly, many scientifically minded physicians have been reluctant to term any test or treatment "futile" or even "marginal." There is, after all, nearly always the chance that a given treatment may help. Screening tests may be too sensitive or insufficiently specific; borderline results need to be re-examined and lab tests need to be repeated.

The ethical bottom line is this: The profession has failed to set its own firm medical standards about what is accepted, proper testing and treatment, and what is not. We often have tested and treated just because the patient or her family asked for it, or about it. **We have generally said "yes" to patient choices, letting them become an expensive proxy for genuine patient autonomy, which isn't the same thing.** The result has been runaway health care costs, and a loss of control to managed care, medical administration and practice guidelines.

Many practice guidelines used by managed care organizations are actually written and updated by Seattle-based Milliman and Robertson, an actuarial firm that interviews experienced managed care physicians and managers about cost-effective practices and treatments. Kaiser, Cigna, Prudential and many Blue Cross/Blue Shield plans use the standardized Milliman guidelines, either adjusting them to fit local conditions, or using them straight from Seattle, according to the *New York Times*.

Milliman says its guidelines are written for non-Medicare patients who are under age 65 and do not have complicated courses or conditions. Utilization managers use the guidelines to reduce admissions, lengths of hospital stays and services. Guidelines are currently written for inpatient, outpatient, home health and back-to-work care; dental and pharmaceutical guidelines are pending.

As a medical ethicist and a professional chef, I know that "cookbook medicine" is no better than the recipe writer and tester. Cookbook publishers contractually obligate cookbook authors to test their recipes before they are published. Shouldn't guideline writers be similarly obligated? Shouldn't practicing physicians know if guidelines save money or improve quality, and if so, with which ingredients and in whose kitchen?

Quality has many definitions. It is not, however, simple compliance with practice guidelines. Physicians who follow these recipes will burn dinner once a week, and their patients may go hungry. Yet guidelines present an important way to share knowledge, create better practices and keep physicians up to date. And guidelines and physician adherence to them are here to stay.

Plans that enforce practice guidelines as a standard of quality must do so with the participation of front-line physicians. Patients caught by guidelines that are unfair or that do not permit exceptions will hire attorneys to appeal the denial of care. And patients whose attorneys talk to hospital risk management departments for them usually get what they want, even if they don't sue.

Defining quality and goals

We should define quality positively, perhaps starting as quality guru Avedis Donabedian did—structure, process and outcome. Or perhaps we should build on what the RAND Corporation's Medical Outcomes Study has done, with **its seven components** of quality: financial accessibility, organizational accessibility, continuity, comprehensiveness, coordination, interpersonal accountability and technical accountability.

Yet ethics is missing from these definitions. Did the RAND authors just forget about patient values, preferences and choices? Shouldn't these determine the goals for a particular patient's care? And shouldn't physicians have incentives for meeting these goals? Most physicians would be glad to discuss the realism and reasonableness of a patient's goals for treatment. Such discussions would avoid allowing "perceived quality" to substitute for the real thing.

Building patient goals into the definition of quality, and giving patients new chances to consider goals that enhance quality of life as well as survival is the right thing to do, and it's also likely to be the economical thing to do. Who knows? **Maybe we can define quality as that which achieves the patient's reasonable goals.** Now that would be ethical.

Adapted from La Puma J, Hickey M, "Managed Care Medical Ethics: Physicians as Partners," in Hickey, M (ed), Learning to Manage Care: A Basic Science Primer of the Skills and Knowledge Required to Work in Managed Care Delivery Systems. The American College of Physician Executives, in press, 1998.

For Further Reading:

1. Nash IS, Nash DB, Fuster V. Do cardiologists do it better? Journal American College of Cardiology 1997; 29:475–478.
2. Quality improvement without borders. The Joint Commission Journal on Quality Improvement 1997; 23(1)(whole issue).
3. Topol EJ, Califf RM. Scorecard cardiovascular medicine: its impact and future directions. Annals of Internal Medicine 1994; 120:65–70.

6

Managed Care Needs the Credibility of Professional Moral Standards

M ANAGED COMPETITION and managed care are, at minimum, a phase through which the American health care system must pass. The ethical principle of the 1960's, '70s, and '80s, patient autonomy, will merge with the principle of the 21st century: proportionality, or fairness. But are patients, managers and physicians ready for this? Consider two sets of facts.

According to InterStudy, more than 45 million people are now enrolled in HMOs, a 10 percent increase over 1993. An average monthly HMO family premium was $395.94; a single person's was $145.63.

In fall 1994, *American Medical News* reported that Maria Warne of Boise, Idaho, was awarded $26 million on July 20, 1994. Her husband was refused a liver transplant four years before, as transplant coverage was allegedly excluded in the Warnes' HMO contract, but included in an informational brochure describing covered services.

What do these facts tell us? Regardless of their health plan or premium, patients often do not accept tragedy as a part of life. The yellowed death that too often comes from liver failure may be an unpreventable tragedy. But preventable tragedy is evidenced by the nearly 40 million people who have no insurance. They cannot afford to belong even to a managed care plan, with all its faults and constraints.

Those fortunate enough to have insurance may have a choice of plans. Employers often include clarifying data sheets about their offerings, comparing HMO with IPA with PPO with fee-for-service plans. How ironic and tragic that these comparison sheets may someday wind up as exhibits too, as some poor widow or widower pleads a postmortem case on the basis of misinformation or plain fraud.

Some patients will have a shot. They'll be the articulate, aggressive and careful ones, the ones who can use an appeals process, or the ones whose physicians have time and skill enough to help patients appeal, even if it is expensive. But most patients won't have such luck. This is the new twist on the concept of proportionality. HMO enrollees will depend upon a physician's professional moral standards for achieving medical goals.

Collective character

A professional moral standard is built on individual actions and collective character.

It is learned not at a mother's knee, but as part of the socialization of a profession and as part of a community.

How we act when no one is looking, when no one will be the wiser, is shown with patients in the community—in managed care's case, a community of covered lives.

What are some effective, practical steps a physician can take to become a more *personal* physician, one who includes the underserved and models the virtues necessary for patients to succeed in managed care? Here are seven places to start:

1. **Negotiate more.** Identify areas of red tape and solicit the patient's help in breaking through. Keep straight with the patient the difference between what is medically indicated and what is financially available.

2. **Keep medical records.** Document the complexity and intensity of your discussions of patient values, care outcomes and

quality of life. These discussions are essential to good decision-making, and ones in which patients want to participate.

3. **Make the managed care contract explicit to patients.** Urge patients to write to their human resources department to include quality of coverage as well as its cost.

4. **Learn your colleagues' approaches to problems.** Seek simple reports of how many consultations colleagues obtain for the same patient condition, or pool expertise with colleagues to develop collective quality-improvement measures.

5. **Schedule more time for medical and financial discussion with patients—and bill the payer for it.** Inform patients of your constraints and obligations—both avoidable and unavoidable ones—and of the impact they have on your practice. Disclosing financial conflicts doesn't make them disappear, but it is one step toward providing better information to patients.

6. **Urge the individual patient to be an active part of a community.** Find innovative ways to have patients teach each other—for example, through group educational sessions for patients with the same condition.

7. **Use new communication strategies to boost satisfaction.** Patients often want information as much as decision-making authority. Use newsletters, mailings and CD-ROM sessions to patients' advantage.

Management's responsibilities

What responsibility has managed care management to serve underserved patients, and to what moral standard should it be held? Should it be held to the lowest moral standard—the written contractual standard known as the law—or to a higher one? Physicians seek the healing, healthful good of medicine. We're trained with health as a goal, physicians practice daily, and know that they must overcome obstacles to achieve good.

To make managed care go, management must be newly responsive and service-oriented, just like physicians. Plan leadership should do six things:

1. **Consider its geographic community as part of its commitment to health care, especially those members who are underserved.** This is part of what it means to seek health for a community, and it is consistent with a commitment to the welfare of others. It is also easy to pilot.

2. **Demonstrate respect for physicians' professional dedication to care for the sick.** By providing more time to physicians to fulfill professional commitments with educational allowances and updated training for new skills, plans take seriously the professional ethic.

3. **Refute cost containment as the *mantra* of managed competition.** Managed care has been tainted by cost containment as a primary driving force. Focusing on providing access to new populations—the medically indigent, the elderly and minorities, for example—will help to erase that shadow and with luck and hard work, replace it with an image of quality and support.

4. **Invite broad participation in policy-making**, not only by physician-managers, but by front-line generalists. Seeing the dilemmas daily can have rewards at the policy table for a whole population.

5. **Value and pay generalists well**. Current income levels are a major source by dissatisfaction, and physicians, like others, tend to do more of what they're paid well to do.

6. **Acknowledge dual role conflicts**. Treating patients medically and managing resources wisely may often conflict. Repeated, clear identification of conflicts will be necessary to reduce and eliminate them.

For Further Reading:

1. Annas GJ. Patients rights in managed care—exit, voice and choice. New England Journal of Medicine 1997; 337:210–215.
2. Friedman E. Managed care, rationing and quality: a tangled relationship. Health Affairs 1997; 16(3):174–182.
3. Mark T, Mueller C. Access to care in HMOs and traditional insurance plans. Health Affairs 1996; 15(4):81–88.

7

Integrity in Managed Care

Mrs. Goodwin is 42, has been infected with H.I.V. for four years, and is asymptomatic. She has just landed a new job as an office assistant, and is seeing Dr. Beale for a pre-employment physical and a screening mammogram. Mrs. Goodwin's new company does not pay for the physical and her HMO does not cover annual screening mammograms.

Mrs. Goodwin's exam is completely normal, except for mild fibrocystic disease bilaterally. The pre-employment form asks Dr. Beale if the patient has any serious medical problems.

"Doc, do you have to write that I have H.I.V.? I can do the job."

"Ummmm . . . ."

"Also, about the mammogram . . . Can't you write that I have a lump or something?"

FOR INDIVIDUALS, **integrity is a virtue. For organizations, it is a business necessity.** Integrity and honesty go hand in hand, and in managed care, too often the hand has been faster than the eye. Health plans on the top floor of a six-floor walk-up without an elevator may not be illegal, but they aren't exactly poster boys for good behavior.

Integrity is what patients expect from health plans, and integrity is what they will seek, regardless of whether they have to go to regulators to get it. But patients are worried about the fracture of honesty and truthfulness in medicine—can't physicians do something?

Indeed they can. Managed care can care more than it has *if physicians drive the care*. The most important ethical issues in managed care are access and coverage. Here, more is better. Spending prudently on most of us should allow all of us to access coverage. That is the promise of managed care, especially capitated managed care, and it is still possible.

How have organizational integrity and values changed in the era of managed care? Are they fundamentally and deliberately stronger, more virtuous and personal, more open and community-minded? Or have they lost their way, their relationship with their communities, their openness? Do organizations genuinely care about clinical ethics (clinician-patient interactions), business ethics (payer-customer interactions) and social ethics (community-citizen interactions)? If they do, how do they show it?

How has integrity been managed?

Integrity unifies a sense of duty to others with proper business conduct. Though it is rising fast, it has been in short supply in managed care.

Many in medical ethics have also taken integrity for granted and have associated fraud with the unethical research values of the second World War, applied even in peace time, and with the 1940s Tuskegee experiment on African-American men with syphilis, who were intentionally left untreated. In the middle 1960s, Henry K. Beecher wrote that integrity served as a reliable means of self-policing the profession and guarded against future abuses.

Problems posed by physician self-referral and ownership of laboratories and investments in the 1980s, however, and the current corporatization of health care make clear how badly integrity has worked as an ethical self-defense for medicine in this century. **But integrity is now organizational, not just personal, and that is the change in integrity in managed care.** As the delivery of care has been integrated with its financing, patients have come to expect that their physicians are no longer in charge. At least not by themselves. A health plan's billing and informing practices and a health system's conduct that patients read and hear about are what represent a physician to prospective patients.

Some plans go an extra mile—literally—into the community to find patients who miss appointments chronically. This is laudable and good, and it is also good business. After all, a shuttle bus to the office is a lot cheaper than an ambulance to the emergency room, whether for a crisis or for what should be an ordinary primary care visit.

Health care organizations are moral entities. They exist to take care of people, just as physicians do, and have moral responsibilities to patients, families and clinicians in addition to the fiduciary ones they have to shareholders or bondholders. Physician-ethicist Linda Emanuel of the AMA has written that because health professionals are accountable to business values, including efficiency and cost-effectiveness, businesspersons should be accountable to professional values, including kindness and compassion.

In theory at least, business ethics actually has the same sort of standards as medical ethics, with principles and codes. **Business' ethical obligations are integrity and honesty. Medicine's are those, plus altruism, beneficence, nonmaleficence, respect and fairness. Like medical ethics, business ethics regards the law as a floor for ethics—it is the least anyone should do.**

Business ethical issues have always been a consideration for managed care, though as in medical practice and research, sometimes not quite enough. Fraudulent billing, upcoding and unbundling, kickbacks, ownership deals, economic credentialling, and patient dumping between hospitals and in long-term care are at the top of the heap. There is no telling what is at the bottom. These issues are why many people think of "managed care and ethics" as an oxymoron.

This does not have to be. Managed care must clean up its organizational act, and it needs tough new public standards to do it.

As in medical ethics, teaching others *how* to think about ethical issues is more important than teaching *what* to think about them. As in medical ethics, the black and white answers are few and relatively far between, though for issues of integrity, fraud and abuse, there are some obvious dos and don'ts.

Most physicians would never consciously compromise an individual patient's health for a financial reward, but some would and have. Anyone who watches "20/20," "60 Minutes," or "48 Hours" knows that some physicians can be bought. Most physicians know that these few impostors are bad apples that would spoil the barrel and must be tossed.

Such colleagues may be dishonest or simply selfish, but they do all physicians a disservice with their actions. Any harm they cause to patients also harms physicians. A group's and plan's system of policies and processes should protect each physician compelled by conscience and medical practice to defend the medical interests of his or her patients by reporting unscrupulous medical money-making behavior.

Physicians know these ethical questions exist in the profession, but they seem impossible to answer, much less control. They also seem irrelevant, as many employed physicians always feel as if they themselves are one step away from unemployment. Physicians are less satisfied than ever with capitated managed care, though once they get the hang of it, and learn that it is a system that they can make work without systematically sacrificing quality, satisfaction goes up. One group of Kaiser Permanente physicians recently accepted 10 percent longer hours at the same pay so more visits did not have to be crammed into the same hours and so no one would lose his or her job.

But make no mistake: Deselection isn't pretty. It comes suddenly, like a sharp Chicago wind at the end of March, when the lions have re-emerged to search for lambs, who are suddenly silent. **At the moment, deselection can happen to anyone at any time for nearly any reason.** That's why it is so unsettling. Gag clauses, intrusive to begin with, staining and dirty at the end, are almost preferable to physicians: At least gag clauses say what they mean. Non-compete clauses often accompany gag clauses: Physicians who offend the powers that be get 30 or 60 days notice and, once fired, cannot set up practice within five or 10 miles. So, if a medical group or health plan or HMO can disable you anyway, then what does it matter whether a gag clause is in or out? It doesn't.

What physicians really want is long-term financial security—not the huge dollars necessary for loan repayment or a down payment on a dream house. Financial security and job security are not the same things, and both are needed. Long-term financial security has to do with sweat equity and earning a regular paycheck; job security has to do with the possibility of being locked out of the profession while being trained, available and willing.

Will more physicians drive cabs or become lawyers? Probably not yet. There is still the feeling among physicians that patients will always need allopaths, as patients have for more than 150 years in the U.S. **But physicians will need to learn new skills—how to read contracts and negotiate carefully; how to work well in teams; how to evaluate how much profit fairness allows; how to pool physician wisdom and ingenuity and draw from it; how to draw the reward of self-esteem from the relational stimulation and society of medicine.** Clinicians should make sure they are doing what they love, and if not, should find something they do love and do it, perhaps on the side at first, where pure joy can be compensation enough.

Some of that joy will spill over into the next day, and any physician's ability to recognize ethical issues in the office, clinic and nursing home will double. Not surprisingly, they're often business ethics issues.

Should a family physician inflate a diagnosis of diabetes IIB to diabetes IIB with peripheral neuropathy because a 77-year-old man wants to talk about whether he should switch to a Medicare HMO, and needed five more minutes? Should a nurse practitioner upcode a young man's macular truncal lesion by adding a family history of melanoma to the medical record to assure he reaches the

dermatologist? **Should a general internist do a pap smear and endometrial biopsy on a woman with irregular, intermittent bleeding when a gynecologist gets the same capitation rate with little or no difference from the risk pool?**

Issues like these illustrate outpatient clinical ethics. The physicians need enough flexibility and support to say "No" to each question above. Will they get it?

Ethics consultants and committees are sometimes available to help. When they are compensated to consult in patient care, they do so, often with excellent satisfaction ratings. But consultants and committees usually must donate their time to do ethics and too often are isolated, and have little clinical authority and minimal synergy with other institutional programs. This is because no one wants to pay for ethics until trouble comes along.

The best known and best funded ethics programs are the ones created because they were federally mandated by a branch of the U.S. government. These are not token departments to be trotted out at ceremonial events. They are serious, comprehensive efforts, often focusing not on ethics but on legal compliance and standards of business integrity. This is a place to start, but not to end.

To do good in managed care, ethics consultants and committees must know both the business and clinical issues. If bioethicists are not directly involved in patient care, they should be. Physicians should tell them about capitation and conflict, about rationing resources and risking compensation, and about clinical problems of access and coverage. If they are worth their pay, bioethicists will be available to colleagues and patients to help create fair, responsible ethical guidance for tough cases, to appeal decisions when necessary, and to work with utilization and quality management.

Quality in managed care is too often ordinary courtesy and honesty translated into claims for superior service and satisfaction. Here are some truisms about quality: No one knows how to measure it well, or who is accountable for it, but everyone knows it should be maximized, risk-adjusted, reported to the public and of low cost. Plans should compete on it and physicians should be judged on it. It is not "perceived"; it is proven.

What's missing from this is who should help shape it. Quality of care is not a business matter—it is primarily a medical matter. Just as physicians helped society get into an overspent, overbuilt, overutilized rut, physicians should help society get out.

By creating coherent, evidence-based practice guidelines to rate quality, both front-line and management physicians can remind themselves of logical next steps for treatment. Fewer smokers, hyperlipidemics and diabetics slip through the cracks if a guideline mandates screening and a systematic system is set up. Fewer perimenopausal women go without considering hormone replacement therapy and annual mammograms; fewer men go without daily aspirin and regular exercise.

Integrity in managed care: the road ahead

"What do you think I should write?" Dr. Beale asks. "We don't want you to get fired, but I don't want to lie to your company. About the breast lump, either."

"Hmmm—don't you have something you write for everyone?" Mrs. Goodwin asks. "What they care about is whether I can work. I can work. The rest is none of their business."

"You have no medical conditions that compromise your ability to perform the job. That's true. We can write that. But if I say you have a mass and the truth is you really can't afford it, then what?"

"Doc, I don't know. Why don't you just tell them that, then?"

Dr. Beale calls the HMO for permission to order the screening mammogram, but the line is busy twice, and once he is put on hold for what seems like forever. His assistant reaches an authorizing nurse on the fourth call. The nurse promises to fax the appropriate form for submission and review.

For patients to believe that they can receive honest, personal care from someone they trust, integrity in medical care should be championed by physicians. The idea of an organizational role for physicians is not new, but it has a new force and relevance.

Improving access and choice, seeking honorable physician relations, overhauling billing, coding and referring systems, addressing moral and quality concerns head on—these are the actions that can restore managed care's tarnished credibility. Physicians are part of this system. They could help improve it—a lot.

What can clinicians do to bolster organizational integrity and maintain their own?

1. **Take on a part-time management position.** It can be as simple as sitting on a management committee or doing the office's claims to ensure accuracy and improve cash flow. Become part of a medical group with a cooperative culture. Learn leadership skills: It is survivalist and worthwhile.

2. **Ask for an ethics mechanism to address hard choices:** an expert outside panel for disputes about medical necessity; an alliance with an independent bioethicist or the local hospital ethics committee chairman to see patients or come to meetings when needed; an indigent patient fund to pay for those whose care is medically needed but financially unavailable; a research partnership with a health plan or sponsor to answer relevant questions about health care services.

For Further Reading:

1. Miller TE. Managed care regulation in the laboratory of the states. Journal of the American Medical Association 1997; 278:1102–1109.
2. Jecker NS. Business ethics and the ethics of managed care. Trends in Health Care, Law, and Ethics 1995; 10(1/2):53–55.
3. Mariner WK. Business vs. Medical Ethics: conflicting standards for managed care. Journal of Law, Medicine and Ethics 1995; 23(3):236–246.

8

Ethical Issues in
Outpatient Managed Care

IN MANAGED CARE ORGANIZATIONS (MCOs), ethical dilemmas occur in the office and clinic, not just the hospital. Dilemmas are less often about whether to liberate a mechanically ventilated patient whose family wants "everything done" and more often about who among us can prescribe expensive medications for heart failure or anemia; whether to fudge a referral form for a young attorney-patient eager to see the dermatologist about a not-so-new facial nevus; and whether to complete a handicapped-parking permit or sign a home health form for a patient you've never seen, but who has left a message, as you are her primary physician. Outpatient care (and the ethics thereof) is rooted in disease prevention and health promotion; it relies on enrollees sharing risk, and on physicians looking out for a population as a whole; and it seeks to provide care that is necessary, appropriate, prudent and effective.

Outpatient clinical ethics has three major subsets: conflicting loyalties, communication, and professional and social responsibility. Like most clinical ethical difficulties, problems in these areas can be approached most efficiently by learning the details of the case. Here are several clinical ethical concerns in each category:

1. Problems of conflicting loyalties

Financial conflicts of interest. Although physicians have always had to be wise stewards of resources, they have not previously formed partnerships with hospitals and payers to deliver care. Some physicians have found it difficult to be a patient's primary advocate while also a partner of these other parties.

A plan's withholds from physicians, its coverage policies and its financial incentives to limit treatment represent the greatest threat to many patients—and to many physicians. But which financial conflicts distort judgment? Is it fair for a patient with liver cancer to use $200,000 for a transplant, while DEXA scans for bone density costing more than some enrollees can afford, are sometimes denied? Explicit discussion of these conflicts by physicians in the MCO board room is essential for fair resolutions.

Referral and consultation. In MCOs, physicians are advocates for their patients in the examining room, in the waiting room, and on their panel—all at once. When a new patient with tuberculosis receives a referral to his long-term, out-of-plan pulmonologist, it means that a primary physician has found that either the necessary expertise is not available in the plan or, in very rare cases, the physician-patient relationship has therapeutic value that would be lost if a change in physicians were compelled. All enrollees foot the bill. When is such an out-of-plan referral justified?

Legal obligations. Physicians are often caught between utilization management and a hard place. Legally responsible for patient care, they're also bound by the rules of their MCO and often by practice guidelines. Utilization management and malpractice prevention also may collide, as physicians seek to practice defensive medicine, even while acknowledging that doing more procedures does not prevent lawsuits; indeed, only better communication with patients does that.

2. Problems of communication

Disclosure of treatment limitations. Who should tell whom, and how much? Should the plan disclose treatment limitations through patients' employers? Should physicians inform each new patient, or each old patient at every visit? Or should physicians not discuss plan limitations at all, referring patients to the medical director or plan administrator? The doctor's obligation is to recommend appropriate treatment, to help the patient investigate reasons for constraints on treatment, to explain likely consequences and how to appeal the constraint.

Advance directives. The Patient Self-Determination Act of 1990 requires MCOs to inform patients of their right to refuse treatment and to have an advance directive. Patients who have advance directives usually want to discuss their personal values and decision-making, and physicians have the moral responsibility for initiating this discussion in the office.

In the debate about advance directives and euthanasia, patient autonomy and cost containment may be too easily conflated. Honest, careful advance planning may indeed save 3 to 4 percent of health care costs annually. While this is of interest to policymakers, the reason to ask about patients' choices and reasons is because it will help doctors do the right thing for patients, not simply because it may save money.

Cultural diversity. Managed care has traditionally drawn from the white middle class, which has a Western set of expectations and mores about health providers and about what causes illness, disease and symptoms.

What an ethical awakening is coming! As millions of African-Americans, Hispanic-Americans and Asian-Americans enroll, and as the poverty that afflicts immigrant groups comes with them, how will managed care respond? Two issues arise. First, these minority groups have a disproportionately high incidence of expensive illnesses such as AIDS and coronary disease. Will these patients have to pay more? Will managed care reach out with case managers and basic screening? Second, these groups' cultural beliefs about health care often are different from those of middle-class white Americans. Will managed care attempt to integrate these differing social and ethnic traditions? Will it guard against discrimination of all kinds? Will it bring all community members under its tent?

3. Problems of professional and social responsibility

Resident and student education. As part of training, some faculty physicians allow residents and students to make mistakes, e.g., to perform unnecessary physical exams or order inappropriate lab exams. Teaching faculty who balance potential patient discomfort and harm with the professional responsibility to teach students must now include a new obligation: to use the MCO's resources wisely. Will enrollees pay for a faculty member's time to instruct others in the practice of medicine? Is physician training a public trust for which MCOs should be responsible?

Community and public health. The average American diet is 34 percent fat. While patients are not at fault for colon cancer and heart disease, many scientists believe these and other "lifestyle" diseases are preventable. Spending more dollars on the medical treatment of these diseases means fewer dollars to teach enrollees to eat right, to exercise and to reduce stress—and that's a loss for the entire managed care community.

Finally, what is the community in managed care? Is the managed care community one of covered lives? What obligation is owed to the geographic community in which the office or clinic is located? Should the community stick together over time, and if so, how much time?

Is plan cost shifting to cover indigent care obligatory or just warranted? Are membership-only HMOs justifiable when working men and women, downsized out of affordable health insurance, wind up sick and waiting at a county hospital, uncertain of whether Medicaid is available and, if it is, whether they qualify? Is a tax cut for families with children worth a cut in Medicare, and worth each member's new nine-month mandatory commitment to a Medicare risk plan? How much financial incentive does it take to underutilize service and distort clinical judgment?

Unfortunately, bioethicists seldom have put ethics and economics in the same sentence. Ethics problems at the end of life affect, at most, all two million people who die annually in the U.S. But 150 million people are, in some way, in managed care and over 41 million lack access to any care, managed or unmanaged. HMO strategic planning, Medicare reform and capitation negotiation present basic, still unanswered ethical questions.

Patients are experts on the personal, social and familial aspects of their own cases. Physicians are experts on the available medical facts. Together, patients and physicians can approach the new ethical dilemmas of managed care compassionately and responsibly.

Adapted from La Puma J, Schiedermayer DL, "Outpatient Clinical Ethics," Journal of General Internal Medicine, 1989; 4:413–420.

For Further Reading:

1. Council on Ethical and Judicial Affairs, American Medical Association. Ethical issues in managed care. Journal of the American Medical Association 1995; 273(4):330–335.
2. La Puma J, Schiedermayer DL. Outpatient clinical ethics. Journal of General Internal Medicine 1989; 4:413–420.
3. Weiner JP, Parente ST, Garnick DW, Fowles J et al. Variation in office based quality. Journal of the American Medical Association 1995; 273:1503–1508.

9

Anticipating Managed Care's Effect on Culturally Diverse Populations

NEW IMMIGRANTS to the United States are entering managed care. Who are they? What are their values? How do we anticipate the care they need and the issues it raises?

So far, enrollees in managed care organizations have been predominantly middle-class Caucasian, paralleling the physician supply. In 1990, 83 percent of U.S. physicians were Caucasian. By the year 2000, however, the proportion will be 75 percent, and by 2010, 68 percent. Traditionally left out of health care have been African-Americans, Hispanic-Americans, Asian-Americans and Pacific Islanders, and these groups are growing. In the 1980s the number of Hispanic-Americans nearly doubled, to more than 22 million. Asian-Americans are among the fastest-growing segments of the population. The (Southeast Asian) Hmong people, for example, numbered 90,000 in the United States in 1990, a more than 2,400 percent increase in 10 years.

New populations of both physicians and patients will have new expectations, especially about limitation of treatment and care near the end of life. And their assumptions about the value of autonomy, decision-making and confidentiality may not be Western at all.

Culture and Western ways

Patients use culture to understand, interpret and explain their symptoms. Imbalances of body temperature, blood level and social discretion may, for some people, define normal and abnormal. Disease cause, treatment, severity and prognosis may be explained using scientific reasoning and the germ theory of disease—or, instead, by traditions, rituals and beliefs.

In just 30 years, Western attitudes about end-of-life care and truthtelling have reversed from scientific secrecy to talk-show openness. We now believe in the primacy of patient self-determination; in telling whatever we know to the patient (and documenting it well); and in ethical innovations, such as informed consent forms and written advance directives. We emphasize individuals rather than families. Especially in middle-class, urban, industrial America, family is something people are born with and into, not of and for.

Yet non-Caucasians, even while living in Western society, often maintain different values. In a 1993 study [Journal of Clinical Ethics, Summer 1993:4(2);155–165], Caralis and colleagues found that significantly more African-Americans and Hispanics than whites wanted their doctors to keep them alive no matter how ill they were.

Blackhall and colleagues found that Hispanic-Americans and Korean-Americans more often wanted a family member to make decisions for them than to make decisions themselves. [Journal of the American Medical Association 1995;274:813–819]

After practicing medicine for four years on a Navaho reservation, Carrese found that **86 percent of Navaho health providers and patients disapproved of and disagreed with the federally mandated Patient Self-Determination Act—because they believed that telling a patient who is ill and burdened that he or she may refuse treatment would be likely only to bring on pessimism and loss of hope.** [Journal of the American Medical Association 1995;274:826–829]

Managed care connections

Because poverty and ill health are still so strongly correlated with being nonwhite, and because the new enrollees in managed care will increasingly be nonwhite, managed care faces enormous cultural barriers. Will peoples so consistently disadvantaged and underserved respond willingly to managed care limits when they have not received their due to begin with? Not likely. And nonwhites are disproportionately expensively ill.

Just look at the data. The mortality rate for heart disease in African-American males is twice that for white males. Fifty percent of all AIDS cases in the U.S. occur in people of color. One-third of all neonatal deaths are in African-American infants, but only one-sixth of infants born in the U.S. are African-Americans. Hispanics have three times the incidence of Type II diabetes as do non-Hispanics, and diabetic retinopathy is the leading cause of new blindness in the United States.

Managed care organizations that try to accommodate, culture by culture, the values, lifestyles and family relationships that characterize their enrolled minority populations will attract and do right by them. How? Sociology 101 can help. An obese, first-generation Hispanic-American woman with hypertension, for example, does not need to be handed a diet of rigatoni with low-fat cheese and a vegetable stir fry. She needs someone to take the time to find out where, when, how and with whom she cooks and eats.

At its most generous, managed care is a philosophy of public health and population-based care that seems foreign to many Americans. Culturally diverse care needs time and attention, and patient values are a critical part of population-based care. If providers are given sufficient time to pay attention to a patient's social and family history, cultural diversity can be construed not as a barrier to decision-making, but as a practical tool.

An ethics committee role

Care near the end of life and managed care will be important new areas of needed expertise for institutional ethics committees. To understand cultural diversity and to help patients and institutions, clinicians and ethics committees must go to the patient's side and understand the issues that pose concern.

To practice more effectively in culturally diverse managed care:

Emphasize personal respect, using proper family names, and promptness.

Use nonfamily interpreters when possible. Personal conceptions of what medical signs and symptoms mean can be too sensitive to convey through close relatives.

Know that exceptions make the rule: not every Native American will regard a trance as a blessing, and not every Hispanic-American will look at obesity as a sign of prosperity and health.

Ask patients, especially indigent Hispanic- and Asian-Americans, if they want to know their diagnoses and make decisions, or if they'd like someone else to do so. That way, decisions can be autonomous and fair.

Adapted and excerpted in part from La Puma J. "Cultural Diversity, Medicine and Medical Ethics: What are the Key Questions?" Bioethics Forum 1995;11(2):3–8.

For Further Reading:

1. Hamilton J. Multicultural health care requires adjustments by doctors and patients. Canadian Medical Association Journal 1996; 155:585–587.
2. Murphy ST, Palmer JM, Azen S, Frank G, Michel V, Blackhall LJ. Ethnicity and advance care directives. Journal of Law, Medicine, and Ethics 1996; 24(2):99–107.
3. Pachter LM. Culture and clinical care: folk illness beliefs and behaviors and their implications for health care delivery. Journal of the American Medical Association 1994; 271:690–694.

1 0

Medicare in Managed Care: Seeing Patients as "Losses"

EDICARE PATIENTS who enroll in managed care plans present special ethical dilemmas. **It is not just that many Medicare patients are old and chronically ill. It is that capitation for their care places many physicians at greater financial risk than does capitation for the younger, healthier population that many commercial HMOs have carefully recruited.**

Two key ethical issues in Medicare managed care are *underwriting* **and** *the cost of care near the end of life.* These may seem more like regulatory issues than ethical ones, but the problems they pose have unexpected effects on physicians' ability to help Medicare patients achieve their goals. They also illustrate the major ethical problem in all of managed care: how to balance what is financially available with what is medically needed.

Underwriting

Underwriting is an insurance term. It is defined as the process of selecting risk. Health insurance underwriters (insurance agents) attempt to recruit as many healthy people as possible and to avoid recruiting sick people. Insurers aim to lower claims expenses and to achieve higher profits for shareholders. "Cherry picking," "skimming off the cream" and "adverse selection" are industry jargon for some of the most aggressive underwriting strategies.

Insurers aim to minimize their expected patient care costs, or "loss ratio." That's why managed care underwriters may avoid recruiting enrollees in nursing homes or long-term care facilities. Instead, managed care organizations recruit older people in restaurants and hotel ballrooms, attracting the ambulatory elderly. Such patients are often concerned more about overtreatment than undertreatment. They are perfect Medicare managed care enrollees.

Physicians are familiar with the perverse financial incentives that pervade Medicare contracting. But underwriting by managed care organizations is something physicians seldom see or directly experience. And underwriting affects costs, profit margins and patient care as much as price, utilization and other controls on physicians.

Ethical issues raised by underwriting include the language we use to talk about patients. It conveys our attitudes, feelings and values as much as what we say. Physicians have an understandable aversion to referring to patients as "customers," a term that connotes products and transaction instead of professionalism and autonomy. But talking about patients as "loss ratios" is beyond the pale. Is the proportion of illness to profit too high? Whose loss is this, anyway? And referring to healthy people as cherries to be picked and cream to be skimmed characterizes sick people as so much spoiled fruit and sour milk, waiting for the sanitation workers on their weekly rounds.

A second issue is managed care access, limitations to it, and discrimination against people without it. Why should the elderly, often unaccustomed to doctor-shopping and asserting their rights, be unable to access what could be a wonderful system for them—preventive services so they can live longer, with limited costs so they can live better?

Medicare patients should be able to enjoy the real benefits of managed care (prevention and promotion), and will often survive long enough to do it. These patients are older precisely because they are survivors and do not keel over easily. Yet Medicare patients take more medication and have more illnesses than non-Medicare patients, and sicker patients in managed care organizations are often thought of as undesirables and members of the lowest caste.

The end of life

Much has been made of the cost of Medicare. It is projected to cost the federal government well over $200 billion by fiscal 2000, a price tag that is certain to go up in the coming years. The program currently covers about 40 million people, fewer than 10 percent of whom are enrolled in managed care plans.

Care near the end of life is expensive in part because no one can accurately predict when the end of life will come. The necessarily retrospective figures are so controversial and are calculated in so many ways that they are not worth repeating here.

Until recently, most Medicare managed care risk plans lost money. With carve-outs such as the old-old (those over age 85), pharmacy plans, hospice programs and a new clamping down on hospital utilization, Medicare administrators and entrepreneurs now hope to make money—in a hurry.

Medicare patients whose claims are denied cannot appeal them to local health maintenance organization medical directors because these authorities may simply be unavailable. Patients can appeal claims for denied services and unpaid claims to the government's agent for appeals:

David Richardson
President, Network Design Group
1000 Pittsford Victor Rd.
Pittsford, NY 14534

The key ethical issues are these: How much is an older person's survival worth relative to his or her quality of life? To the expense of treatment? To the other potential uses for those resources, including caring for younger persons who may live longer? Is future life to an older person less valuable than future life to a younger person just because it's likely to be shorter? Does the value of life already lived count in how we allocate Medicare dollars in managed care? Should a 71-year-old with Class IV heart failure be able to weigh hospitalization and home care independent of their cost, or should cost be part of that individual's considerations?

The answers to these tough questions are changing. And there's another consideration. When Medicare patients are underdiagnosed or undertreated, the problem affects women disproportionately, because most elderly people are women. Discrimination against them occurs even at the end of life.

Medicare managed care is increasingly attractive to physician managers and executives as risk contracting rates have a high profit potential. Yet as risk sharing becomes prevalent for primary physicians, the financial risk of caring for a generally elderly population can too easily be confused with the medical need to discuss quality of life and survival. Learning about underwriting techniques and about new documentation guidelines are two ways to keep your head up in Medicare managed care.

For Further Reading:

1. Callahan D. Controlling the costs of health care for the elderly—fair means and foul. New England Journal of Medicine 1996; 335:744–746.
2. Donnelly WJ. The language of medical case histories. Annals of Internal Medicine 1997; 127:1045–1048.
3. Miles SH, Weber EP, Koepp R. End of life treatment in managed care—the potential and the peril. Western Journal of Medicine 1995; 163:302–305.
4. Perls TT, Wood ER. Acute care costs of the oldest old: they cost less, their care intensity is less, and they go to nonteaching hospitals. Archives of Internal Medicine 1996; 156:754–760.

11

Informed Consent: Should Capitation's Financial Incentives Be a Part?

APITATION asks doctors to shoulder financial risk for their patients' care. Capitation is defined as a flat "fee per head per time": usually dollars per member per month. Capitation dollars are revenue, which is different from income. Income is what the doctor keeps after paying for health care services.

Bonuses and withholds are common incentives for both salaried and capitated physicians, and also for chief executives. *American Medical News* recently reported that chief executive officer Norman Payson of Healthsource Inc. was paid a base salary of $387,000 in 1994. Yet performance incentives brought his income to $14,280,000. But we are doctors, not executives.

In capitated managed care, and especially in global capitation, the doctor who takes home more does so by spending less on patients. With just this conflict in mind, the Health Care Financing Administration's new rules on incentives limit the amount of potential physician bonuses to 25 percent.

Financial incentives

Should doctors disclose to patients the financial incentives they face to limit treatment? If so, should this disclosure be part of informed consent discussions?

Financial incentives in managed care are not new. Patients have them: to stay in network, to use the formulary, to avoid durable medical equipment, to question experimental treatment, to defer cosmetic and alternative treatment. Patients who do these things usually save money.

Physicians have financial incentives too—to limit testing and treatment. Rewards go to physicians who limit referrals, stay within formularies, lessen laboratory use and reduce average hospitalization to 200, 180, and even to 150 days per 1,000 members.

Financial incentives to limit treatment that result in less care for the patient and more reward for the doctor represent an acknowledged conflict of interest, even if less treatment is better, and if the doctor's financial reward is a coincidence. But does this conflict of interest sometimes distort sound judgment or result in patient harm?

Distorted judgment

Financial incentives *should not* be allowed to distort judgment. Our historic tradition as an altruistic profession is strong. Physicians in the United States have a ritualistic focus on the individual. Threats of malpractice litigation and the law loom if we do too little. Hospitals and payers police care already and will catch us if we slip. And of course, many physicians do not know, for example, how much ten days' worth of clarithromycin actually costs.

But financial incentives can distort judgment and sometimes do. Nearly everyone has a price for which he or she would, other things being equal, make decisions that err on the side of keeping 10 percent, 25 percent or 100 percent of income. This is not a moral flaw, but simply human behavior. Doctors are not different from other workers: We do more of what we are paid well to do.

There are at least three ways to attempt to minimize the possibility of distortion: informed consent, disclosure and regulation.

Informed consent

Informed consent is information, understanding and noncoercion. The information must be adequate for patient decision-making; the understanding must be genuine, and not simple reiteration; and the decision must be volitional. The most important reason for applying informed consent is to protect patients against any unwanted treatment and its potential risks.

Financial information is not currently part of informed consent, perhaps because conflicts of interest do not present a risk of treatment, but instead, may simply warn people about the limits of their doctor's loyalty. Yet the risk of distorted judgment is the risk that patients take in capitation.

Disclosure

Disclosure to patients is difficult and may be ineffective. The financial incentives that affect physicians' choices depend in part on the amounts of money involved, and different patients have different ideas of how much money is a lot. The doctor-patient exchange has power and knowledge on one side, and need and fear on the other. And few patients want to choose between accepting their doctor's prescription and pondering his motives.

On the other hand, **disclosing conflicts of interest to patients may increase trust and meet an objective test of what a reasonable patient should know.**

Regulation

Regulation may also help minimize the distortion of judgment. For example, we can:

- decrease how often bonuses and withholds are given
- create a large minimum for the number of physicians sharing in the reward

- create a large minimum for the number of patients for whom physicians are responsible
- increase the time between feedback reports to physicians about financial performance

Discussion of financial incentives to limit care should move out of the shadows into the bright light of doctor-patient dialogue. To preserve trust, and show that physicians are patient advocates, they should tell patients how they are paid, and how managed care payers restrict and encourage them. They should do this because it is honest, because patients want to know, and because patients believe in the goodness of their own doctors. The information is also available in *Newsweek*, *Vogue*, and *USA Today*, and on the nightly news and the Internet.

Disclosure of financial incentives, however, is not an office procedure to be performed while examining the breasts of a 45-year-old whose mother died of cancer or the heart of a 55-year-old whose cardiomyopathy has led to failure.

Instead, **honesty should be an office policy. Physicians can use simple, one-page handouts about what managed care is, how it works, and how offices are reimbursed.** Physicians should **emphasize their first loyalty, but note that they too have to live within the rules,** and that they are learning about this new system, just as patients are. **They should use appeal processes when a patient's personal medical interest is at risk.** Fortunately, not every patient will need an appeal, perhaps only one of 50 or even 20, among the chronically ill. They should be able to present appeals in policy settings—in board rooms, medical director meetings, and top management forums.

It is patients to whom highly paid executives must respond. It is, after all, patients' money.

For Further Reading:

1. Hillman AL, Ripley K. Physician financial incentives in managed care: their impact on healthcare for the elderly. American Journal of Managed Care 1995; 1(2): 199–204.

2. Meisel A, Kuczewski M. Legal and ethical myths about informed consent. Archives of Internal Medicine 1996; 156: 2521–2526.
3. Morreim EH. To tell the truth: disclosing the incentives and limits of managed care. American Journal of Managed Care 1997; 3(2):35–43.

1 2

Bound or Gagged?
Privacy, Confidentiality
and Computerized
Patient Records

CONFIDENTIALITY in managed care is not a misnomer, but it is in question. Confidentiality usually in-
volves keeping private any information learned from or
about the patient. It can sometimes be ethically breached, and in
some cases must be—suspected child or elder abuse, gunshot or
other suspicious wounds, communicable diseases, and workers'
compensation cases.

Some managed care issues concerning confidentiality
are new. First, people in private organizations, not just
government, may newly discover and use information not
meant for them. Second, the computerized patient record
(CPR)—which despite its initials does not need to be re-
vived so much as to be buttressed with RAM (random
access memory)—makes an order-of-magnitude difference in information access and the potential for breach.
Third, some physicians are required by contractual agree-

ment to keep information *from* the patient about therapeutic options, or about their health plan.

Keeping secrets

Many patients recognize that a distant episode of depression requiring hospitalization, once recorded under their "Past Medical History," may brand them for life with an employer or insurer. So, a terminated pregnancy may not be volunteered, and hence not recorded, in the "Review of Systems" or in the "Past Surgical History." Notice of a single episode of later-in-life syphilis or several youthful homosexual encounters may also never make it to the doctor, much less into the medical record.

To gain access to managed care, prospective utilization review asks patients to be forthcoming about their physical and mental problems. To avoid embarrassment and maintain privacy, some patients avoid making a necessary appointment with the triage nurse or social worker. Others, cowed by the process, minimize their symptoms.

To intrude into a person's privacy, the state must show a compelling interest, writes Galveston attorney William Winslade. To learn confidential information—information that was once private—the state must show logical reasons. Private companies, however, have no right to such data, yet may seek it.

For example, in the case of *John Doe v. Southeastern Pennsylvania Transit Authority* (WL 683382 U.S. Dist. Ct., E.D.Pa. 1994), a patient's employer was found liable for inappropriately using knowledge gained by evaluating an employee's prescription, written for treatment of HIV disease. The employer had allegedly received the prescription information from Rite Aid Corp., a pharmacy chain. Another lawsuit, this one filed against Rite Aid, was settled out of court in favor of the employee.

The trouble with computers

How many times has a doctor had to see a patient and not had the records? Were they checked out to the hospital four months ago?

Or were they here just yesterday, only to be moved on to the department in charge of quality improvement?

Computerized patient records are supposed to change that trail, and with luck they will. Complex patients can have records three feet thick. Even three inches is impossible to review in a 20-minute office visit that may begin, "I just have a cough . . . and need some prescriptions refilled." Wouldn't mouse clicking and 17-inch monitors be easier?

They probably *would* be easier for everyone. **But federal protection of electronic information is largely nonexistent.** Scores of people and institutions can now know whatever doctors know about the patient, whether or not doctors or the patient approve.

There are programming-based tools for protecting information. Encryption is one; read/write limitations are another. There are also responsibility-based tools, such as passwords and audit trails.

Yet all have problems. Passwords, for example, can be copied, lost, stolen or just happened on. Their existence can allow users to be distant or remote. Users may hurry off to the next patient and become remote, forgetting that they've logged in, allowing ready access to anyone who walks by.

A quivering lip

Gag rules take many forms, but most prohibit physicians from discussing diagnostic, therapeutic or consultative options not covered by the patient's managed care organization. Many prohibit discussion of the plan's referral procedures, including financial incentives and utilization penalties for physicians.

At least five states (Colorado, Maryland, Massachusetts, Oregon and Tennessee) have passed laws limiting or quashing gag rules. And legislation in the House of Representatives would outlaw gags in contracts and fine managed care organizations that fired or refused to pay a physician who spoke with a patient about the risks and benefits of tests, referrals or treatment.

Disclosure and trust are the foundation of any potentially therapeutic relationship in health care. Neither exists if the doctor cannot speak about the quality, relevant outcomes and experience of the health plan. There is little debate about these points.

What there is debate about is what constitutes a gag. Does it include "anti-disparagement" clauses, in which the physician promises not to malign the managed care organization with patients or colleagues? Do physicians know how different plans work well enough to explain them?

There is also little recognition of a safety gag—our collective reluctance to write something in the chart because of the patient's shame or confidence, or feared unemployment or divorce. Sometimes a safety gag is made explicit by a patient's quivering lower lip or explicit request or both.

What is a doctor to do when a patient asks to keep something off the record? It's easy to say that under most circumstances, private information linking patient and condition should not be revealed without a patient's specific permission. But, knowing as we do that perfect confidentiality is hard to assure, when are we justified in omitting pertinent information from a patient's medical files?

Most physicians have acceded to requests to leave out, say, an HIV test requested after an episode of unprotected heterosexual sex that the patient wants to keep secret. But the waters rapidly become murkier if one moves on to the suppression of more clinically significant notations like alcoholism, drug addiction and abuse, and sexually transmitted disease. Lying to protect patients can only be a temporary solution: in the end the disease and the deception will come back to bite both.

For Further Reading:

1. Bayer R, Toomey KE. HIV prevention and the two faces of partner notification. American Journal of Public Health 1992; 82:1158–1164.
2. Farber NJ, Berber MS, Davis EB, Weiner J, Goyer EG, Ubel

PA. Confidentiality and health insurance fraud. Archives of Internal Medicine 1997; 157:501–504.

3. Gostin LO, Turek-Brezina J, Powers M, Kozlorf R, Faden R, Steinauer DD. Privacy and security of personal information in a new health care system. Journal of the American Medical Association 1993; 270:2487–2493.

1 3

Confidentiality Again: Drug Plans Need an Ethics Infusion STAT

PRESCRIPTION DRUG PLANS are an attractive feature of many managed care organizations (MCOs). These plans may be a bargain for patients who need very expensive medications, such as Foscarnet to suppress CMV retinitis ($2,300 for 30 days, wholesale to the pharmacist). But for other patients who need routine meds, some prescription plans are a rip-off.

Prescription plans and formulary committees are under fire. As at least one prominent MCO reported a $70 million surplus in 1994, patients and physicians have financial as well as moral grounds to demand better service and a fairer approach. At least four major ethical issues arise: subsidies, titles, access and theory (STAT).

Subsidies

In a Sept. 27, 1994, letter to *The New York Times*, Harvard Medical School's Richard Spark, M.D., wrote that one HMO charges $15 per 30-day prescription for thyroxine, as it does for all other medications. This works out to $180 a year. The HMO honors only one prescription per medication per month. The retail price of a 12-month supply of thyroxine in Boston is between $65 and $88—*half* of what this HMO's enrollees pay.

In addition, Sparks wrote, the HMO restricts its enrollees to filling their prescriptions at the pharmacy chain CVS to "guarantee a constant monthly flow of traffic to CVS, with the expectation that subscribers, while waiting for the pharmacist to put 30 pills into a vial, will roam the store, purchasing toothpaste, hairspray and shampoo, thereby further increasing the revenue of CVS at the expense of the subscriber."

Should HMOs effectively subsidize pharmacy chains with the prescription fees of enrollees? Should patients know that their $15 monthly fee pays for both their thyroxine and their neighbor's Foscarnet? Should a physician help a patient to appeal these arrangements on behalf of the patient who needs thyroxine?

Titles

In this context, titles mean patient names and conditions. The dilemma is how to keep them confidential. Sadly, no longer is information learned from or about the patient safe with a doctor. Others, including those trying to pay or adjust a claim or verify enrollment data, have reasons to want to know the information.

Confidentiality has been termed a decrepit concept, and the law has been called upon to provide a floor through which confidentiality cannot fall. For example, **a Pennsylvania patient's employer was found liable for inappropriately using HIV prescription information against the patient.** The employer had allegedly received the information from a pharmacy benefit management company. The employee's lawsuit against the company was settled out of court, in the employee's favor.

Other ethical issues range from whether to make drug utilization and health benefit records available to employers, regulators, researchers and others who may have claims to the information; whether a physician should be able to insist on brand name medication, and if so, who pays the difference if a less expensive brand or generic equivalent is on the formulary; whether an MCO may reject payment for a drug when its efficacy and safety are uncertain; and how to keep a computerized drug information system safe and private.

Access

Should MCOs microallocate resources by permitting only certain physicians to prescribe expensive drugs? Is this morally justified for any medications?

Perhaps. If overused, new antibiotics lose some of their power and organisms develop resistance. Infectious disease specialists, able to keep track of the differences between myriad cephalosporins and mycins, may be well suited to hold the keys to state-of-the-art expensive antimicrobials.

But the same justification cannot be offered for limiting primary care physician and patient access to antianginals or antihistamines or botanicals. Is this strategy for reducing use of expensive, sophisticated medications just a way to reduce a MCO's costs? By discounting patient convenience, MCOs may force primary physicians to refer to a specialist, just for a prescription. And no primary physician can justify that—to his or her conscience, to utilization management or to the patient.

Theory

The theory behind prescription plans, like much of managed care, is noble: Disease prevention and health promotion strategies are likely to improve quality of life, extend survival and keep patients where they'd rather be—at home and out of the hospital. Providing the medications that patients need at a fixed, modest price facilitates health promotion. Patients want the best medication and take it for granted that physicians will prescribe it.

Yet as more patients with fewer resources have greater access to managed care, managed care organizations ask, "Is the best drug necessary here?" if the best drug is an expensive one.

What is the "best" drug, and when is it needed? If a drug kills 97 percent of isolates, instead of 92 percent, can be taken once daily instead of three times, and often causes no side effects, instead of occasional nausea and vomiting, is it not a better drug? If it is a better drug, isn't the other one nearly as good? And if it is nearly as good, does that justify "therapeutic substitution" by a pharmacist? Or by the physician?

Should the physician tell the patient that the best drug is actually not needed, and that the second best (which happens to be on the formulary and is much cheaper) will probably be adequate? Should the patient be given a choice—in the medical office?

Prescription slips

Only 70 percent of prescriptions are filled, and compliance falls as dosing frequency rises. When MCOs limit patient and physician access to medications, patients may have to forgo treatment, or pay out-of-pocket for medications that should be covered.

Keeping straight the differences between what is medically indicated and what is financially available is the central issue in managed care ethics. Physicians have enough to do already in managed care, but administrative action is needed to help patients. We must demand open disclosure about prescription plans, and then help to educate our patients about them. We should applaud better and more open disclosure about MCO arrangements with pharmacies. We should explore whether two-tier prescription plans have a moral basis.

Patients often expect prescriptions when they visit their doctor's office and many patients leave the office holding one. By clarifying the details of prescription plans, physicians can make sure that prescription slips are worth the paper they're written on.

For Further Reading:

1. Gray BH, Perreira KM. Medical professionalism under managed care: the pros and cons of utilization review. Health Affairs 1997; 16(1):106–124.
2. Soumerai SB, Lipton HL. Computer based drug-utilization reviews—risk, benefit, or boondoggle? New England Journal of Medicine 1995; 332:1641–1645.

PART II

14

The Principle of Beneficence in Managed Care

Mrs. Chilaca is 67 and has severe peripheral neuropathy from diabetes. She has tried tricyclic anti-depressants, massage, narcotics, anti-inflammatory agents and anti-epileptics. Her granddaughter recommends rolfing, a form of massage that tears connective tissue, and she has been to a chiropractor for several adjustments, without success. She takes only metformin and glyburide.

Her examination shows hairless lower extremities below the knee, poorly palpable dorsalis pedis pulses and absent posterior tibialis pulses bilaterally. Her shiny smooth skin is insensitive to touch or pain. There are no cracks between her toes.

Her glycohemoglobin was 6.7 percent two months ago.

"What about hot peppers?" she asks Dr. Beale. "My granddaughter says they help the circulation—all I do is dry and blend them in a blender to make a liniment. Or how about if I just added some salsa to my eggs in the morning? Yum!"

BENEFICENCE means doing good. Before managed care, responding to "medical indications for treatment" meant an urgent, immediate, rule-out, disease-centered response. Medically needed data motivated testing and procedures. Beneficence meant doing more.

At its most thoughtful, managed care understands physicians' duties to do good differently. Imagine you're on the banks of a river, and all of a sudden fully clothed people bob past, all swimming to reach shore. Instead of just pulling people out of the river downstream, managed care reasons, why not go upstream and see why they're falling in?

How has doing good changed in the era of managed care? Do medical indications for diagnosis and treatment still come first in decision-making? If not, then what is the touchstone for knowing how to act? Can a physician do good for a group of people whose apparent unifying characteristic is that they found his or her name in a book?

How, then, has the principle of beneficence been modified by managed care?

The change in beneficence in managed care is **that doing good is no longer just a disease-centered effort. Instead, it is person- and population-centered,** and because it is both, it is tricky to master. Physicians have always wanted to do good for individuals and groups, but their inquiry has sometimes been scientifically driven more than personally driven. The goal, of course, is to do good for an individual patient and for the population of which the patient is a part. The trick is to motivate patients to care enough about themselves and their families so that they want to prevent health problems in their communities.

Beneficence in managed care is customer-focused, cost-conscious and flexible. **It asks physicians to help whole populations avoid expensive treatments when possible and to emphasize basic cost-effective treatments. Doing more is out; knowing how much to do is in.**

To do good in managed care, physicians must develop the conviction that some new matters of public health belong as part of ordinary medical practice. Physicians will have to help patients to educate themselves and take a bigger decisional role in their care. In short, **beneficence will look a lot more like self-help than paternalism. And in most cases, it should.**

What are the other cases? **Those of patients who cannot act for themselves, who are on the margins of the system, who are uneducated or illiterate, who need special care. For these patients, clinicians cannot afford to let self-help carry on by itself.**

Doing Good in Practice

Doing good for patients usually has more to do with *process* **than outcome, and it takes time. And skill.** Often it is not the clinical decision itself that is most important to patients, even those without decision-making capacity, but the way in which the decision is made, including who makes it. The families of patients in persistent vegetative state, for example, may surely have different personal agendas than the patient might, but just as surely have moral authority to ask for closure.

In negotiating with such families, and attempting to do good, physicians are allies with other clinicians such as pharmacists, who have been effective, unpaid patient advocates for as long as the corner drugstore has compounded pills, powders and elixirs. Pharmacists are subject to some of the same rules and incentives that guide and push physicians. As the corner drugstore morphs into a drug information and counseling center, pharmacists will be primary patient educators—to patients' advantage.

Doing good has never included gaining access to futile treatment. The ethical arguments about futility are much ado about very little. It is financial arguments that matter about futility.

The real point about *futile treatment* **is to identify it before it is instituted, clarify its medical uselessness, and help patients escape it.** Here is an issue on which clinicians and managed care can readily agree: Treatment that is neither medically effective nor personally beneficial has no business being administered, is wasteful and often can be prevented.

Unfortunately, futility now is being defined by employers, market forces and legislators. Payers are deciding what is futile treatment, and patients are screaming. Legislators have heard their screams, and in 1997, more than 1,000 managed care bills were introduced in state legislatures and over 100 in the U.S. Congress, where a health care "bill of rights" is being debated.

Inappropriate and futile treatment would rapidly go the way of radiotherapy for tonsilomegaly if medicine would publicly define futility's medical boundaries. But medicine has not. For example, a 52-year-old woman comatose for four years develops stage IV pressure ulcers. An internist refers her for wound healing and surgical repair. A surgeon makes the repair. If a physician will do it, and an insurer will pay for it, then neither medicine nor managed care has decided it is futile.

Physicians should be willing to be clear about what works and what does not—and stick to their guns. If medicine is to be shaped by a commercial ethos and defined by efficiency, then the least physicians can do is to be medical and scientific, and let legislators fume about the consequences of studied, unified medical judgment.

Gatekeeping has become the art of persuading the patient that he or she does not want what he or she cannot have. Yet few physicians believe that the monies saved by using appointment delays and a third selective serotonin reuptake inhibitor (SSRI) instead of psychotherapy will create better access to care for those with no access. Creating access to care for those with no access is the true purpose of gatekeeping and using resources prudently, especially in capitated managed care. It is yet to be realized.

Something negative like gatekeeping *could* be turned into something positive, like becoming a hospitalist and creating new flexibility for medical practice. Patients gain a skilled, focused, available additional doctor. For increasing numbers of primary care physicians and multispecialty groups, *a hospitalist is an efficient inpatient colleague co-attending the patient*—not a house physician in-house only long enough to put out fires and get enough sleep to go to his or her real job the next day.

Fortunately, gatekeeping is likely to become history as both patients and physicians tire of micromanagement. Direct access to specialists will be more the rule than the exception. Giving patients the tools to prevent disease will become the primary care clinician's job. Though educational disease prevention tools may seem medically marginal, patients do not necessarily view them as such.

Marginal treatment **itself is often subjective and necessarily case-specific, and like futility, is neither an entitlement nor an obligation.** With pre-managed care concepts of beneficence, the physician sometimes did more to make sure the patient or family knew no stone had been left unturned, swearing under his or her breath the whole time. No one *needs* marginal treatment. In fact, not only is marginal treatment unlikely to help, it is sometimes unwanted. And *providing* unwanted marginal medical treatment is more likely to result in a lawsuit than is *withdrawing* unwanted marginal medical treatment.

Doing good for patients with alternative or complementary medicine is still quackery for a minority of physicians, and a routine inquiry for another minority. An estimated $20 billion 1998 market, approximately 75 percent of which is paid for out of pocket, is now going to health food and grocery stores, chiropractors, herbalists, acupuncturists and energy healers.

Even with all that cash going elsewhere, managed care is not eager to embrace all nonallopathic clinicians, especially those who are unlicensed. There are precious few controlled trials of alternative treatments. There are even fewer practice guidelines available to tell a general internist when to refer a patient with acute back pain to a chiropractor, or an HIV-infected infant to a touch therapist, or a nauseous pregnant woman to an acupressurist.

Integrative medicine, which combines allopathic and nonallopathic treatments, represents an underacknowledged way to do good for patients. Those physicians who can find out what is effective and safe and what is not, and who begin to integrate some of the techniques, procedures and medications that help and do not harm patients can serve them, both as individuals and as a population. Learning about alternative medicine is good service, and deserves front row interest by physicians.

Customers expect a service orientation at Nordstrom's, the

Ritz-Carlton, Brennan's and Tiffany's. But is medicine enough like retail to say the customer is always right and buyer beware? Should physicians offer a money-back guarantee? Is this a good thing to do in health care, or an impoverished way to think of doing good?

Professional ethics has always encouraged patient service first, beyond anything required by ordinary courtesy, and certainly beyond that required by law. A service orientation is second nature to physicians, but medicine is not the same as commerce. Money-back guarantees give back only money, and it is health and empathy that most people really want.

The beneficent answer? Principled stands against tobacco, violence, and wanton profiteering. Principled stands for better pain relief, better access, uniform cholesterol screening, more screening mammograms and mandatory seatbelts and helmets. Accountability and incentives for physicians doing their part, and for patients doing theirs. Practice ethics by principle—no exceptions.

Beneficence in managed care: the road ahead

"Hmmmm . . . chilies. Capsaicin is the chemical that makes hot peppers hot," Dr. Beale says. "It's over the counter in a 5 percent cream. Use gloves. Put it over the whole area at least three times every day for four weeks. Don't touch your eyes, nose or mouth afterwards. Be careful—it stings at first. You don't have to dry and powder chilies yourself—you'll never know how much you have, and if you inhale the stuff we may have to put you in the hospital."

As capitated managed care grows, physicians will become responsible for keeping members healthy, not just taking care of the sick. Doing good sometimes means balancing the health of a population against the needs of a single individual. This is a precarious, unforeseen balance that no physician relishes, and it is only defensible if an opportunity exists to do good for the whole panel or population.

"Rescue me" is how we've done good up until managed care. "Teach me to swim" is what's ahead. But right now, there are a lot of people in the water, and more falling in all the time. That's the immediate problem. And managed care companies that wish to distinguish themselves from the competition have to pull people out and provide incentives for wellness.

What can clinicians do about promoting wellness when so many are sick?

1. View beneficence as a way to reinforce patients' ability to decide for themselves—not the nurse's, physician's or manager's ability to decide for them, especially about wellness and lifestyle issues.

2. Participating must be linked to deciding. Ask patients to bring blood pressure logs, blood sugar logs, exercise logs and diet logs to the office. Write agreed-upon "quit dates" for smoking in the record. Ask those who can to participate more in their own care: clinicians are not there just to pick up the pieces when patients go into renal failure, develop claudication or become ketoacidotic. Clinicians are there primarily to prevent those problems.

3. Offer to give a public lecture for the hospital or community or church group. Choose a subject that is important to many patients—vaccinations, hormone replacement therapy, cardiac or neoplastic disease. As much as possible, let audience members teach each other.

4. Approve, empathize, and as appropriate, express concern or worry in the office. Make sure people feel cared about. Do these things instead of approving, appealing or ordering treatment that is unlikely to be medically effective or personally beneficial. Try to offer evidence-based explanations.

5. Embrace medicine that works safely and reject medicine that does not, regardless of what it is called. Speak out against quacks who would dupe patients with unsubstantiated claims. Recommend and learn alternative medical methods that demonstrate effectiveness and safety.

6. Involve patients by involving the whole team. Skilled, educated, motivated, trusted team members will want to innovate and improve the practice. Who in the office radiates a can-do cheerfulness, or a constructive know-how? Who can take on

a mini-research project on great teaching materials for patients, or find community organizations willing to meet the office halfway? Who can set up your office web site?

These suggestions can help bring physicians and patients closer. Managed care can facilitate that by:

1. creating individual smoking cessation, seatbelt and cholesterol report cards;
2. making evidence-based medicine an operating strategy for utilization management;
3. educating physicians about alternative medicines and technology by using traditional forums such as continuing medical education conferences, books and newsletters; medical grand rounds and teaching conferences; and journal clubs.

For Further Reading:

1. Alper PR. Learning to accentuate the positive in managed care. New England Journal of Medicine 1997; 336:508–509.
2. Kassirer J. Managed care and the morality of the marketplace. New England Journal of Medicine 1995; 333:50–52.
3. Reinhardt UE. Wanted: a clearly articulated social ethic for American health care. Journal of the American Medical Association 1997; 278:1446–1447.

1 5

Should Doctors Guarantee Results? Or, Whose Disease Is It, Anyway?

P HYSICIANS know that grades are coming—for number of patients seen, length of hospital stay, formulary compliance and patient satisfaction. But it is not only managed care plans, patients, physician groups and state agencies that grade physicians. It is also the marketplace.

In medicine-as-free-market twist, **Massachusetts has now made public its physicians' malpractice histories for the price of a toll-free call.** The office handling the calls reported receiving more than 500 in the first day of operation.

In a parallel twist, other physicians are responding to market demands like marketeers. The Pacific Fertility Center promises that if, after it makes two treatment attempts, a woman doesn't have a pregnancy that lasts at least 12 weeks, Pacific will refund 90 percent of the fee that covers its medical services. The fee does not cover medical screening, medications, other medical services or "egg donor agency fees."

Ethics for sale

To make matters worse, Pacific says its "ethics advisory board, made up of independent, internationally acclaimed bioethicists, has judged the IVP [in vitro fertilization partnership] Plan to be highly ethical." I wonder if my colleagues donated their services to Pacific, or charged only a nominal fee, for surely it would otherwise be difficult to make an independent judgment about this extremely complex problem.

Even ethics has a price

Public use of doctors' malpractice histories and of money-back medical guarantees is emblematic of the new consumerist face of medicine. Health care is a service, this face says, and it should be selected and evaluated like plumbing or heating—caveat emptor. Advertisable outcomes matter most.

If a double dose of hormones is necessary to effect ovulation, and it also happens to effect a hyperstimulation syndrome, Pacific doesn't cover it. And if a malpractice suit against you arrived after your weeks of struggle to save a very low birthweight baby, it is on your record.

Outcomes like suits and guarantees are conspicuous, but they are not the whole story. They oversimplify the complex and reduce process and experience to a single metric.

Yet many Massachusetts callers want to know everything they can about their own doctors before they visit again. They probably like the proof of quality that a money-back guarantee furnishes for consumer goods such as toaster ovens and frying pans. Don't we all? If there were a refund available for unsatisfactory office visits, don't you think people would take it?

Medicine, however, is different from toaster ovens and frying pans. The power and trust physicians have built individually with individual patients cannot simply have vaporized. If medicine has changed to "buyer beware," is the change permanent? Should the ethics of the marketplace replace the ethics of the profession?

Pediatrician and ethicist John Lantos of the University of Chicago has argued that patients expect miracles because medicine has been so good at producing them and because they occur routinely on "ER," "Chicago Hope" and "Rescue 911." Off the screen and on the cutting room floor lie scattered bits of human tragedy, far more common than successful cardiopulmonary resuscitation.

Expecting a miracle is neither wise nor prudent. Yet physicians will increasingly be held responsible for tangible, measurable outcome assessments in populations that are costly to managed care plans.

Which assessments? Diabetics' glycohemoglobin measurements. Asthmatics' peak flows. Pneumovax vaccinations in your at-risk population. Appropriate mammography and Pap smears. Seat belt documentation in the medical record. Preventable hospitalizations.

"What?" you cry. "I didn't give my patient asthma or diabetes or breast cancer! I just tried to treat it." Or, "I followed the practice guideline our group or the American College of Physicians or another organization created, and the patient still had a stroke or was hospitalized or had a complication."

Tough. The principles of consumerism in managed care mean that your patients should do better than the patients of others— well enough to advertise. If your patients are sicker than your colleague's, then relative value units should show it.

If doctors are to be held responsible for patients' illnesses *and* habits, then whole new seminars in the documentation of patients' missteps, not to mention medical ethics, will be needed. Why? Because now there are other alternative healers coming to the fore. They too see sick people, and many of those people are our most difficult patients—those with pain syndromes and connective tissue diseases, and chronic illness of all types, including ill-defined symptoms that physicians have been unable to name or ameliorate.

Just like physicians, these alternative healers have professional conferences where it is sometimes hard to tell the commercial exhibits from the instructional seminars, but also where therapeutic song and dance are taken seriously. And patients do not seem to be asking for guarantees from these healers—just time, understanding and demonstrated efforts at partnership.

The collective mistrust of physicians as a whole has served to galvanize individual patients into answer shopping, sometimes thought of as doctor shopping. In many cases this shopping is sad, as such patients often do not have a physician they regard as compassionate and do not have a therapeutic relationship with anyone.

Different incentives?

Is there a way out of this mess? **Rewarding physicians for spending more time with patients, instead of less, might go a long way toward reinvigorating the physician's image as a compassionate healer. Financial incentives could exist for other variables, such as achieving quality-of-life goals for patients.** Objectives measured could include pain-free days for cancer and arthritis patients; ratings of personalness in care (which meta-analyses of satisfaction data show that patients value most); and reduction in polypharmacy for long-term care patients.

Though the illness is the patient's, it is the physician's job to help him get through it so that he can do the things he wants to do. **Money-back guarantees give back only money, and it is health and empathy that most people really want.**

For Further Reading:

1. Epstein RS, Sherwood LM. From outcomes research to disease management: a guide for the perplexed. Annals of Internal Medicine 1996; 124:832–837.
2. Gleiner JA. Patients as customers in the ER. The Physician Executive 1996; 22(11):4–8.
3. Greco PJ, Eisenberg JM. Changing physicians' practices. New England Journal of Medicine 1993; 329:1271–1273.

16

Medicine by Legislation: Can Physicians Learn Techniques That Patients and HMOs Already Know?

I N 1 9 9 6 , 3 5 S T A T E S tried to control managed care
with more than 50 bills ranging from maternal length of stay
to grievance procedures to continuity of care. In 1997, thou-
sands of proposed laws about breast cancer surgery and experimental treatment were on the docket. Congress will again get into
the act in 1998, with action on a consumer bill of rights, including appeal mechanisms following prior legislation.

Is the future of managed care medicine more rules, regulations
and laws? If so, shouldn't physicians take a hint from patients and
use the media and our political processes?

Patient protection

Throughout the '80s and '90s, constituency groups of patients
have learned, courageously, to lead with their illnesses, and single-
service mandates are now popular. **Twenty-two states have
passed laws mandating 48 hours of inpatient care for a
vaginal delivery and 96 hours for a Cesarean.** Breast cancer
surgery is likely to be a continuous hot topic in state legislatures.

Bone marrow transplants, coronary angioplasty or experimental procedures may be next.

Unfortunately, even rules designed to protect patients may not work because of what people already know to be true: Some managed care organizations profit by prohibiting access to treatment. In 1996, six states prohibited prior-authorization requirements for emergency treatment or established a "prudent lay person" standard for defining an emergency.

Pain and anxiety—about cost

In my office last month, a 69-year-old woman who had been discharged on a Monday after a coronary angioplasty called the following Saturday complaining of aching in her chest all night. I suggested the need for an ambulance, but the patient's husband objected, saying the trip to the hospital might not be covered by her HMO. He and his wife deliberated for 90 minutes while her pain increased. Finally, after my nurse's third call to her home, the patient was taken to the hospital by ambulance; she stayed three days.

I saw the patient and her husband in the office this week. Her repeat angiogram showed adequate flow and no infarction. She was exhausted, of course, but glad that the trip to the hospital had cost no money.

The "prudent lay person" definition of "emergency" had not yet filtered down to my patient. All she and her husband "knew" was that they had to get permission. That permission meant coverage, and coverage was necessary in case she had a second heart attack. That she really needed my encouragement and not my permission mattered little: **The word has gotten around that managed care organizations might not pay for emergency treatment, even for severe conditions.**

A number to dial

Other new state laws try to protect better-informed, actually dissatisfied patients. California, as usual, is the leader, having passed six managed care bills in 1996, and had many more held up by the governor in 1997. **A new phone number (800-400-0815) con-**

nects patients with a state-created mechanism to appeal
treatment denials. The Department of Corrections—an auspicious title, to be sure—will send out a form for a patient to complete, even before the patient has finished with the plan's
grievance procedure.

Some new state laws protect physicians. Seven states
mandated plan acceptance of gynecologists as primary
care physicians. Fourteen states passed laws prohibiting
HMOs from "deselecting" physicians and others who fully
disclose diagnostic and treatment options to patients.
Three states passed laws to force plans to disclose physicians' financial incentives.

David Himmelstein's groundbreaking "Sounding Board" column on gag rules in the *New England Journal of Medicine* retrieved
the United HealthCare job he had temporarily lost and publicized
the restraints on truth-telling that many physicians had accepted—
until then.

Mum's not the word

In my office, patients often ask what I think of their health plan,
or if their health plan covers this or that, or whether they should
change health plans. I tell them, confidentially. And patients often
tell me what they think of the physicians to whom I refer them.
"Don't ask, don't tell" should not be the rule in patient care.

In the me-too '80s and me-first '90s, altruism and compassion
have had it tough. The big moving forces have been big media:
television, the Internet and the entertainment industry. Unfortunately, "Chicago Hope" and "E.R." act as social change agents as
actively as many physician groups, and more effectively than most.

Bedside physicians have not yet learned to lobby for altruism
and compassion, or for their own fair treatment. Managed care, by
contrast, has learned to lobby for its interests. Rules on physician
incentives and capitation recently issued by the Health Care Financing Administration, for example, are easier on managed care
than the initial drafts that preceded them. Physicians at risk are
those for whom 25 percent of compensation comes from with-

holds and bonuses, and whose groups care for fewer than 25,000 patients. But HMOs haven't won every battle. Witness, for example, the federally sanctioned ability of any plan's enrollees to find out with a phone call how their physicians are paid.

These laws protect groups of patients and physicians from managed care processes widely perceived to be out of an individual's control: utilization management, exclusive contracts, information disclosure, grievance procedures, and plan monitoring.

What doctors need

The new laws suggest that physicians need their old values—medical professionalism—together with new skills—political skills.

Professionalism is one of the reasons that alternative providers are flourishing and can charge undiscounted fees and command out-of-pocket payments. These providers still inspire faith and trust individually and still have the time to talk to patients personally.

Political skills are honed inside organizations: negotiating, goal-setting, understanding someone else's interests and needs and meeting them. In truth, doctors already practice these skills inside academic departments, within medical associations and medical groups, and sometimes at a patient's side. **As medicine is regulated, physicians who have these skills will survive and thrive—and so will their patients.**

For Further Reading:

1. Bodenheimer T. The HMO backlash—righteous or reactionary? New England Journal of Medicine 1996; 335: 1601–1604.
2. Redman BK. Clinical practice guidelines as tools of public policy: conflicts of purpose, issues of autonomy and justice. Journal of Clinical Ethics 1994; 5(4):303–309.
3. Tunis SR, Hayward RSA, Wilson MC et al. Internists' attitudes about practice guidelines. Annals of Internal Medicine 1994; 120:956–963

17

Alternative Medical Treatments Raise Some Ethical Questions

LTERNATIVE MEDICINE is the politically acceptable term for nonallopathic health practices, usually unavailable in physicians' offices or hospitals, that are very
popular among patients.

Alternative medicine encompasses mind-body interaction,
homeopathy, naturopathy, chiropractic, botanical medicine and
more. Diagnostics range from detailed examination of the pulses
and tongue in Oriental medicine to long personal, medical, envi-
ronmental and social histories in homeopathy. Therapeutic
modalities can include art therapy, the postures and exercises of
Chinese tai chi, and the herbs, purgatives and rubbing oils of the
ancient Hindu medical system ayurveda.

Many physicians believe alternative medicine is unproven at
best and unsafe at worst. Stanislaw Burzynski, M.D., has used "an-
tineoplastins" derived from urine to treat some neoplasms, and the
FDA's raid on his Houston clinic and his trial last year were reported in the press. Nearly every physician has a story to tell about
excess radiographs ordered by chiropractors or the wildly varying
quality of botanical medicines.

What issues does alternative medicine present for clinicians?
What ethical questions does it raise? What can we learn from it?

The big question in alternative medicine is "What works and works safely?"

The ethical principle is beneficence, or "How should we do good for this patient?"

Acupuncture is 5,000 years old; the Chinese undergo major operations with it. Self-help support groups plus nicotine patches are a more successful smoking cessation intervention than nicotine patches alone. The University of California Berkeley *Wellness Letter*, a conservative publication, recommends that patients with heart disease ask their cardiologists about Coenzyme Q-10.

To begin to discover what works, the National Institutes of Health's Office of Alternative Medicine, established in 1991, has given more than 40 pilot and nearly a dozen full research grants. Can electrochemical treatment help malignant tumors? Can intercessory prayer ameliorate drug abuse? Are certain Chinese herbs useful in patients with HIV infection?

Research methods in alternative medicine, however, generally do not follow the Western randomized, controlled trial ideal. Many practitioners have been unwilling to subject their therapies to double-blinded analysis. A focus on the individual, along with nuanced variation in diagnosis and therapy, makes the systematic application of the same research protocol to all enrollees seem foreign to many alternative practitioners.

Patient preferences

Consumer interest drives this field. The ethical principle here is autonomy, or "What does this patient want and why?"

One in three Americans reportedly used some sort of alternative therapy in 1990. A 1994 federal law, the Dietary Supplement Health and Education Act, deregulated the sale of herbs, vitamins, supplements and extracts. Now, every Wal-Mart and Walgreen's has racks full of supplements and slips of paper explaining their use. Patients buy them both by the fistful.

Patients prefer "personal" care. But American physicians and medicine as a whole are not viewed as personal. Contrast this with the image of a practitioner interested in

holism and balance, not diseases and drugs. A practitioner who wants to know you and your needs, not just know what you don't have. Someone who will not scoff at your visits to a colonic therapist or think of the 1960s when you mention macrobiotics.

To many patients, it does not seem to matter that alternative medicine's assumptions are not based in Western science or that its methods appear unorthodox. Actually, some of its methods are standard in other cultures. *The Berkeley Wellness Letter*, for example, notes that 15 million Japanese take Co-Q 10 daily.

Contextual factors

The ethical principle here is justice, or "How should we treat this patient, given the needs of others?"

Eisenberg's study ("Unconventional Medicine in the United States," *New England Journal of Medicine* 1993; 328:246–252) estimated 1990 expenditures on alternative medicine at $13.7 billion. Hospitalizations in 1990 cost Americans $12.8 billion.

Most alternative medicine is paid for out of pocket, but managed care is beginning to cover certain treatments and practitioners.

Kaiser Permanente reportedly operates a successful pilot center for alternative medicine in Vallejo, Calif. It offers acupuncture, massage, meditation and yoga.

The state of Washington's insurance commissioner has ordered access to and coverage for visits to "different state-certified providers for treatment covered by their insurer . . . [including] physicians, acupuncturists, naturopaths, midwives, nurse-practitioners, massage therapists and others," according to *American Medical News*. **Washington insurers still pay, even though the commissioner's order has been overturned.**

Reimbursement for services is a very hot button. Nonphysicians have established the market for alternative medicine and want to be included in managed care settings. They argue that many allopathic treatments are also unproven, yet are reimbursed. But which "alternative" expertise is special? Should alternative treatments meet allopathic cost-effectiveness criteria?

Quality-of-life factors

The ethical principle here is nonmaleficence, or "Do no harm," because quality-of-life factors are determined by the patient. The ethical question is "How should we treat this patient so that no harm results?"

Alternative medicine is not always harmless, by any means. There have been reports of deaths from the herb ma huang, an ephedrine-like substance promoted for asthma. *The Annals of Internal Medicine* published a report of four cases of pennyroyal toxicity in 1993, one of which was fatal. Pennyroyal is a sweet-tasting herb with abortifacient qualities.

Prudent practitioners know the power of the doctor-patient relationship and use the trust patients invest to help them get better. Alternative practitioners rely on trust, too. Medicine is a largely self-regulated profession with checks and balances, which holds its practitioners to reasonable medical standards that are socially sanctioned. Can the same be said for alternative medicine?

Physician referral to a stress management expert or biofeedback center does not seem unusual—these centers appear unlikely to cause harm. But who is a reliable hypnotist or an expert naturopath? What are their credentials? When should primary care physicians be responsible for a naturopath's recommendations?

The challenge alternative medicine presents is to find and test those practices that are better than allopathic practices and to integrate these practices into medical care. We can—and should—learn a lot from practitioners who welcome our most difficult patients.

For Further Reading:

1. Brett AS. Relationships between primary care physicians and consultants in managed care. Journal of Clinical Ethics 1997; 8(1): 60–65.
2. Cooper RA, Stoflet SJ. Trends in the education and practice of alternative medicine clinicians. Health Affairs 1996; 15(3): 226–238.

3. Eisenberg DM. Advising patients who see alternative medical therapies. Annals of Internal Medicine 1997; 127:61–69.
4. Moore NG. A review of reimbursement policies for alternative and complementary therapies. Alternative Therapies 1997; 3(1):26–29,91,92.

1 8

Pharmacists and Physicians: Perils, Potential and Parallels

As PHYSICIANS are deselected and de-listed from managed care plans, sometimes without warning or obvious reason, so too are pharmacists. They are being replaced by things they can't see and don't know how to understand, much less stop. Yet there is hope for physicians and pharmacists who believe in patient advocacy and are willing to collaborate and adapt.

Managed care threatens to extinguish pharmacists' relationships with patients and providers. Pharmacists are struggling to hold on to what they treasure most: the ability to talk with patients and counsel them about medication effects.

In days gone by, pharmacists could make pills, powders, elixirs and suppositories. The pharmacist combined his role as a small business owner—available, accessible, and often visible from behind the counter—with that of a health care professional—competent, licensed, self-regulated, and committed to helping patients. No one could accuse pharmacists of being in it for the money. They were lucky if they cleared 2 percent, versus the 15 percent median annual profit rate that drug manufacturers recorded in 1993.

More recently, pharmacists have been transformed from dispensers into clinicians. This is to the good; the

more people with sufficient understanding of a patient's medical condition and personal situation to help, the better. Pharmacy students now train with medical students, and sometimes rotate on the same teaching services. Especially in complex cases, physicians-in-training turn to their pharmacist-in-training colleagues and ask them, in so many words, to prescribe. When older physicians were in training, this sometimes took the form of calculating aminoglycoside dosages. Now physicians ask, "Do we use an aminoglycoside, or other gram-negative coverage?" The pharmacist can tell, and does.

As recently as 1967, codes of ethics forbade pharmacists to discuss with patients the medication just dispensed. To avoid breaching the privacy of the doctor-patient relationship, labels sometimes did not appear on bottles, except in Latin. Yet patients need and want information, sometimes more than anything else— except someone to listen. And so the neighborhood pharmacist fills not only child-proof bottles, but a real need.

Pharmacists listen when no one else will, or can. When people can't get an appointment for a week or two with their primary care physician, many stop by Walgreen's or the corner store and ask for a little informal advice over the counter. And being the compassionate, good souls they are, pharmacists attend and comply. Many pharmacists know their patients and the physicians in town or in the neighborhood well and serve as effective, unpaid patient advocates.

Unremunerated expertise

Unpaid? Counseling time is not in the "fill fee" pharmacists now receive per bottle. Like physicians and everyone else, pharmacists do more of what they are paid well to do. They are not paid by managed care to discuss drug interactions, listen to a customer's complaints about her diabetic neuropathy, or drop off analgesics at a homebound patient's home, as she lives just a mile and a half away. They are paid to put pills, capsules and liquids into containers. And now that job is threatened, too.

Some pharmacists still own their own stores. Even without

the ability to negotiate for discounts with drug manufacturers, providers and employers, some store owners are proudly and nervously holding on. But pharmacy-by-mail services, pharmacy benefit managers and drug manufacturers are all cutting deals and seeking rebates with employers and health plans, and sometimes with each other. And as go the discounts, so go those services that do not seem to make up the revenue discounted. Reading scripts and dispensing advice are two such services.

How much work is it to read a script? **The most common cause of medication errors is human error. Illegible handwriting, misspellings, and inappropriate abbreviations make prescriptions potentially dangerous in a way informed consent can never cover. But an alert pharmacist can catch the error. Approximately 9 percent of all prescriptions are queried, and many of us are thankful they are**—just for the one out of 10, 20 or 100 where we really did make a mistake.

What's the solution to this messy scribble? Software, of course. Imagine looking over a patient's problem and medication lists on your work station monitor, clicking on a list of formulary-approved antibiotics, highlighting one, and telling the patient a moment later, "Your prescription is waiting at the pharmacy." Imagine a drug interaction warning popping up appropriately, preventing harm and malpractice.

No more phone calls to the pharmacy, or being put on hold. No more phone calls to the patient about refills. No more unnecessary person-to-person contact. Privacy? As secure as electronic transmission. Legibility? If you can click a mouse, you can write legibly.

So, will the pharmacist-patient relationship in managed care become, like the physician-patient relationship, more efficient, hurried, and administrative? Will it incur the dual loyalties and financial conflicts of the physician-patient managed care encounter? Will it still have the warmth and personal dimension that only someone you trust can offer? Will its covenant be reduced to a contract, so that pills become widgets and counting and delivering them safely is enough?

Or can pharmacists adapt, and find ways to participate in formulary committees, ferreting out therapeutic duplications and asking the hard questions about why "me-too" drugs are still there? Or why generics are, on average, 31.5 percent cheaper than brand-name drugs? Can pharmacists conduct educational sessions for patients, perhaps using databases to create disease management programs for all patients on insulin in the managed care community?

Can pharmacists become advocates for the cause of access to medication for the medically indigent? How about a second, cheaper formulary—listing effective, proven, late-1980s medications, now very cheap, instead of this year's newer, shinier models? Can pharmacists collaborate with industry to create research standards for postmarketing research, starting with prospective, peer-reviewed, written protocols approved by institutional review boards? Can pharmacists find new ways to keep patient identifiers confidential, so that a patient's AZT prescription does not become an employer's knowledge?

Like physicians, pharmacists can thrive in managed care, but they need colleagues, encouragement and new skills. Physicians should recognize that pharmacists are clinicians and patient advocates too, and often save physicians and patients time and trouble. One good turn deserves another.

For Further Reading:

1. Brody B. Public goods and fair prices: balancing technological innovation with social well-being. Hastings Center Report 1996; 26(2):5–11.
2. Council on Ethical and Judicial Affairs. Managed care and managed care cost containment involving prescription drugs. Code of Medical Ethics: Current Opinions with Annotations, Sections 8.13, 8.135, pp. 126–130. The American Medical Association, Chicago, 1997.
3. Luce GR, Lyles, CA, Rentz AM. The view from managed care pharmacy. Health Affairs 1996; 15(4):168–176.

1 9

What You Should Know About the Role of Hospitalists

MANY PRACTICING PHYSICIANS have moonlighted as a hospitalist or house physician, usually during their postgraduate training. Yet the position of "house doctor" is no longer one for trainees.

The role of house doctor is changing and becoming newly important, as many medical groups and hospitals agree on the need for a designated attending physician for inpatients. The position signified by that title—as an attending physician-partner with other attending physicians—helpfully answers ethical concerns about house physicians' current role. Like the house physician himself or herself, these concerns have gone quietly unnoticed for years.

At least three ethical questions arise for current house physicians and the organizations that hire them: Should the house physician-patient relationship carry the same obligations as any other physician-patient relationship? Should the house physician owe first loyalty to patient, attending physician or payer? And should the attending physician be compensated for the house physician's efforts?

Relationships with patients

Currently, house physicians and attending physicians are seldom members of the same medical group, though often both are medical staff members with hospital privileges and parking passes. House physicians are, as a matter of employment, asked to stand in for the patient's attending physician, and do the routine and urgent things that attending physicians are otherwise expected to do. Admission histories and examinations, for example, are required by many hospitals, as are discharge summaries.

But how should today's house physician explain to the patient the need for a "routine" history and physical exam performed by an unfamiliar physician? Or the reasoning behind a new doctor-patient relationship—an independent relationship to be truncated as soon as the patient is discharged?

In a way, the still prevalent role of the house physician as an independent, hospital-based attending physician surrogate and extender is medicine's equivalent to an employer's frequent change of health plans. Both the house physician's role and the employer's benefit plans are designed for economies of scale, and neither for continuity. Both count on the patient to ask good, focused, careful questions about who will be the patient's doctor, and for how long.

Dual loyalties

Some house physicians are employed by hospitals or health care systems, and others by medical groups. Ordinarily, hospitals provide the house physician's services to medical staff, though increasingly, medical groups and managed care organizations hire a physician or a medical team to manage the group's patients in the hospital. Skills and roles can include critical care management, risk and utilization management, and medical ethics. The quintessential insiders, house physicians remain underutilized in practice.

But for whom does the hospital-based house physician work? Does he or she work for the hospital, carefully documenting the patient's acute condition, forming an independent professional assessment and offering an unsolicited second opinion about each case? Or does the house physician work for physician-colleagues, even if not a member of their group, and pull together the too often disparate elements of any newly admitted patient's care, from counseling worried family members to consulting old nursing home records? Each role probably could be a helpful one. But without a unified system of physicians, hospitals, payers and groups, the two sets of tasks risk being set against one another, to no one's advantage.

Concerns about professional integrity and quality of care raise similar questions of loyalty. **How should a hospital-employed house physician act if he or she evaluates a patient and finds no reason to believe that the patient needs hospitalization? Or that the antibiotics that are prescribed are off-formulary and a very expensive way to treat the patient's sepsis? Or that the patient wants to talk with his or her doctor, but attending rounds are so early or late that patient and doctor always miss each other?**

Does the house physician have any standing to blow a whistle, as an agent of the attending physician whose behavior may be problematic? House physicians with only the same authority as physicians-in-training often have more experience and greater standing in the medical staff and in the eyes of the law. House physicians without the same incentives as patients' attending physicians are caught between quality assessment and their own jobs.

Fair compensation

In teaching institutions, residents perform services, and attendings co-sign their notes and bill for the services provided. This practice is under scrutiny in graduate medical education funding circles and is underlying dramatic change, but the accepted swap has been training and supervision for dollars and service.

House physicians are not just residents any more. Most house physicians take the role of an attending physician extender in both teaching and nonteaching institutions. Licensed physicians in training still may moonlight as hospital-employed house physicians in most states, but fewer opportunities are available for them. The weekly working hours of residents are now limited, and fewer residents are available. To make up for this loss, both hospitals and medical groups increasingly employ one or more salaried physicians to promote management efficiency.

House physicians are still usually fully qualified attending physicians in salaried positions of minimal authority. The little-discussed practice of an attending-colleague double billing a payer for a house physician's salaried service invites invidious comparison with Medicare fraud-and-abuse provisions. In these cases, a careful examination of billing patterns could be too revealing for comfort. Both hospitals and physicians are at risk here.

A new role: designated inpatient attending physician

Ethical issues of relationship, loyalty and money have other important correlates: discrimination, respect and power. Many current house physicians are international medical graduates. Discrimination is rife against both these physicians and their patients—both are likely to be people of color, at the low end of the socioeconomic scale. Respect for patient confidentiality is often difficult to maintain in the hospital, and even more difficult when providers and patients of different and sometimes clashing cultures are involved. Under these circumstances, power is the unspoken turf issue for attending physicians, who have less and less, and for house physicians, who have almost none.

In coming years, increasing attention is likely to be paid to the new role of designated inpatient attending physician, an appropriate one that suggests the house physician's new importance in managed care and the great possibility for physicians who want to improve patient service.

For Further Reading:

1. La Puma J. House physicians: accountabilities and possibilities. Archives of Internal Medicine 1996; 156:2529–2533.

2. Ubel PA, Gould S. Recognizing bedside rationing: clear cases and tough calls. Annals of Internal Medicine 1997; 126:74–80.
3. Wachter R, Goldman L. The emerging role of "hospitalists" in the American health care system. New England Journal of Medicine 1996; 335:514–517.

2 0

What Are the Utilization Rules for Providing Marginal Treatment?

C A R E is never marginal: Physicians can always offer comfort, encouragement and kindness to a patient in need. Treatment, however, may be marginally helpful. Decisions "at the margin" of effectiveness often mean unique, specific clinical judgments for particular patients.

Lori Nolan is a 27-year-old woman with a 20-year history of Friedreich's ataxia and a recent religious conversion to Christianity. Her disease had resulted in quadriplegia, deforming scoliosis and a severe restrictive cardiomyopathy. The patient had put herself through college and obtained a degree in forestry.

She was admitted with respiratory failure and remained mechanically ventilated after a near respiratory arrest. Her cardiologist wrote a DNR order on the fourth hospital day at 5 a.m. "per family," as the patient's father didn't want her to "suffer anymore."

No specific prognostic data about her disease process were found, though data on survival to leave the hospital showed rates of less than 2 percent for patients who, like her, had left ventricular ejection fractions of less than 20 percent. The patient had a tremendous will to live, the cardiologist noted, and might overcome apparently insurmountable odds.

On exam, the patient was awake and alert. She was ventilated but able to nod and shake her head appropriately. She was in atrial fibrillation at a fast rate.

When asked, "Do you want CPR even if you have only a 2 percent chance of surviving?" she nodded her head to indicate yes.

The ethics consultant pointed out that the patient had decision-making capacity and should be asked about medical decisions. He also noted that her family would probably support the patient's decisions, despite their difference of opinion with her.

The consultant recommended that a heart transplant be considered, that the patient's care be reevaluated after a reasonable period of time, and that significant efforts be made to incorporate the spiritual beliefs so important to her in her treatment plan.

Cardioversion of the atrial fibrillation was attempted. The cardiologist decided to resuscitate the patient if she arrested. She survived in the hospital for several more months, and despite several cardiac arrests maintained consciousness and conversational ability before she suffered neurologic deterioration in the last several weeks and died.

Why definitions matter

A marginal treatment can be defined as a therapy, medication or device that offers minimal potential for benefit and effectiveness to a particular patient, given his or her medical condition.

Benefit means meeting the patient's reasonable goals for treatment; effectiveness means achieving the medical and physical goals for treatment. This definition of benefit helps avoid an open-ended entitlement demand from patients; the definition of effectiveness helps avoid unilateral physician decision-making.

Marginal treatments tend to be seen as out of place in managed care organizations (MCOs). Members of MCOs share risk, and when one requires expensive marginal treatment, others are placed at financial risk. Make no mistake: Treatment like that given to Lori Nolan is financially marginal for MCOs and for hospitals.

In Lori Nolan's tragic case, the patient was persistent in saying what she wanted.

Her desire for treatment seemed authentic, deliberate and heartfelt. The physicians, too, believed her treatment should be continued. Patient autonomy and physician beneficence coincided.

Still, there was something missing. Economic considerations were never raised for discussion explicitly. Even though CPR was likely to be on the extreme margin, Lori Nolan was determined, and her 27-year-old body would try not to let her down.

What can physicians do?

When a physician is faced with questions like those in Lori Nolan's case, **the first step is to assess the patient's own choices about "marginal treatment" as part of a relevant medical history.** What chances would your patients, especially those with chronic disease, want to take if they needed a ventilator? Or intensive care? For how long? Why? Or why not?

This assessment takes time and deserves a separate office visit. Ideally, it occurs as part of a history and physical, even if it needs to be divided into two or three sessions. This well-invested extra time is more than repaid in hospital days saved if patients medically require life-sustaining treatment.

Second, provide information to patients about other treatments for their condition. Information by itself may be therapeutic, allaying personal concerns and conveying the sense that the patient has been included in the process of care. Information about transplantation should, for example, be given to a patient with metastatic breast cancer, regardless of whether a transplant in her case is likely to be effective, part of practice guidelines, or covered by her MCO.

So, **when is marginal treatment ethical?** The uncertainty of medical facts, the uniqueness of patients' personal situations and the often unknown nature of patients' own goals make this a difficult question to answer well. Coupled with the need to integrate the decision with the goals of other managed care patients—people your patient usually doesn't even know—the assessment becomes nearly impossible.

Yet if we could change one of those variables—especially our ignorance of patients' goals—**we might say that managed care marginal treatment is ethical (or fair) when purposefully made available by the community as a whole.** This suggestion assumes full participation by community members.

Medically marginal treatment is hard to make rules about. Problems measuring the quality of care and assessing outcomes data make it harder. Value choices should be part of treatment protocols, but patients have such varied information bases and beliefs that they may not yield to a prescriptive policy.

Paying for marginal treatment

In the case of Lori Nolan, the ethics consultant factored in the patient's choices, including devout religious belief and a strong drive to live. Will, determination, vigor and medical uncertainty can combine to defy the numbers—even overwhelming ones.

Too often, physicians may misdiagnose illness or overestimate futility, especially at the margin. These are unfortunate but inevitable mistakes, for which patients should not have to pay. However, wanting an expensive procedure when the survival rate is only 2 percent is a demand that is less acceptable to physicians and to society now than it was in the 1980s.

The physician's ethical obligation is to accept neither an open demand for entitlement to services nor a rigid insistence on medical certainty when such a thing rarely exists. Instead, sharing decision-making with the patient when she is able, and her proxies when she is not, remains the best way to determine when treatment is ethical.

For Further Reading:

1. Mirvis DM, Chang CF. Managing care, managing uncertainty. Archives of Internal Medicine 1997; 157:385–388.

2. Meslin EM, Lemieux-Charles L, Wortley J. An ethics framework for assisting clinician-managers in resource allocation decisionmaking. Hospital and Health Services Administration 1997; 42 (1):33–48.

3. Reiser SJ. Criteria for standard versus experimental therapy. Health Affairs 1994; 13(3):127–136.

21

Needed: Clear Standards for Defining Futile Care

I S FUTILITY A MORAL ISSUE or a money issue? Should morals and money be separated, or brought together? Two recent legal cases give physicians hope and pause.

In March 1995 in Boston, a Superior Court jury needed only two hours to acquit Massachusetts General Hospital and two physicians of malpractice charges. The physicians had written DNR orders for and withdrawn mechanical ventilation from a 72-year-old dying woman in a persistent vegetative state (PVS), despite her daughter's objections.

The jury found that continued treatment would have been futile and of no benefit, and that the orders and treatment withdrawal were justified.

In April 1995 in Seattle, a jury required only four hours to decide that Highline Hospital and its physicians had acted properly when the physicians discontinued nutrition and hydration from a severely disabled man, at his father-guardian's request. The patient had been determined by a neurologist to be in PVS in 1993. The patient's ex-wife had sued, saying that the patient was able to communicate with her by blinking, and did not want his gastrostomy tube and alimentation discontinued.

The importance of these cases centers on how to define and

identify futile treatment. **The key ethical issue they raise is whether ethical and financial concerns should be separated in discussions of futility.** **The issue is similar to that of marginal treatment: whether medically marginal treatment (for the patient) should be separated from financially marginal treatment (for managed care organizations).**

Futility did not become a hot topic until after 1983—when Medicare's prospective payment system was implemented. Prior to that year, futility was hidden behind the shadow of newly constructed hospital towers and surgical suites, and no one talked about it or its costs.

When the financial incentives of fee-for-service care ruled, many scientifically trained physicians felt free to pursue each diagnostic possibility, and were often encouraged by patients and families to do so. In fact, patients and families came to expect more investigation, and equated it with better treatment—even when it could not achieve medical goals, or seemed to effect more complications than benefit.

Physician-ethicist Steven Miles has parodied the costs of providing futile treatment that are still paid by those unwilling to grapple with money and morals. Miles characterizes these costs as "virtual" because hospitals did not complain, "nonexistent" because costs were shifted, and "irrelevant" because of the inequitable distribution of resources within the health care system as a whole.

But with managed care come financial incentives to limit treatments and even undertreat patients, and cases like those in Boston and Seattle. Futility has arrived front and center—and it is an ethical issue, one that was there all along.

Different people define futility differently, depending on their own goals and values. If the goals of treatment are unclear or in dispute, then futility is in the eye of the beholder. If the goals of treatment (e.g., cure, prevention, education, rehabilitation or palliation) are clear and agreed upon at the start, then people can decide with their own values whether a treatment is futile.

Futile treatment is defined here as one that will not be either medically effective or personally beneficial for a particular patient. Effective means "achieves its medical goal in this case." Beneficial means "achieves its personal goal, for this patient and her values." When treatment is truly futile, few patients or families demand it. The exceptional cases sometimes wind up in court, often because of a nonclinical issue. Physician-ethicist John Lantos has written that futility is really about trust, hope and fear—not about medical care.

Patients or families may not trust the doctor or managed care plan to determine what is futile; they may hope what the doctor and plan have said is mistaken; they may fear the consequences if treatment really is futile. When patients lose trust, money or hope out of proportion to what they expect, their feelings of vulnerability and sense of loss can harden into conflict. **In the debate about futility, the determination of who should pay and how different parties should be allowed to participate in the decision to continue or terminate care becomes the real locus of the moral conflict.**

Professor George Annas, J.D., has written, "It is impossible for physicians to argue credibly that treating patients in persistent vegetative states is contrary to standards of medical practice, because most physicians actually provide continuing treatment if the family insists. Treating medical care as a consumer good is a central reason why medical costs are out of control and why a national health plan that gives physicians financial incentives not to treat seems attractive to many policy makers."

Physicians can no longer wait for society to "speak" on these matters. Society does not have a larynx, or post office box or billing address. The health care system of the foreseeable future is managed care. To clearly articulate moral choices, physicians should make the costs of care more evident—both in cases of futility, like the two above, and in other cases as well. Otherwise, the potentially constructive dialogue about which treatments work, which don't, their costs and their payers will be reduced to grumbles about individual patients, middle-of-the-night ethics consults, and infinite academic debates that help no one.

Without clearly delineated medical standards, and with the rising importance of cost containment, the day may well come when regulators and payers, not doctors, decide which care is appropriate in Boston, Seattle, and everywhere in between.

In discussing futility with *patients*, ethical and financial considerations should be *articulated separately* but in the same conversation. In discussing futility *policies*, decisions about who should pay, who does pay, who should be insulated, and who should be exposed are central, and must be *articulated together*.

As physicians look at the ethical issues in managed care—ranging from coverage and informed consent to experimental treatment and community responsibility—we will need to think clearly, out loud and in public about how costs and futility are related.

We must be willing to articulate and act upon the conviction that medicine should not be just another consumer good. Medicine is a personal service of a respected profession with standards requiring the highest ethical behavior. Those standards, together with our medical expertise, form the foundation of what must become clearly delineated medical principles for treatment.

For Further Reading:

1. Brody H, Campbell ML, Faber-Langendoen K, Ogle KS. Withdrawing intensive life-sustaining treatment—recommendations for compassionate clinical management. New England Journal of Medicine 1997; 336:652–657.
2. Caplan AL. Odds and ends: trust and the debate over medical futility. Annals of Internal Medicine 1996; 125:688–689.
3. Lantos JD. Futility assessments and the doctor-patient relationship. Journal of the American Geriatrics Society 1994; 42:868–870.

22

Assisted Suicide and Managed Care: Whose Right to Die?

P OLLS consistently show that 60 percent of the American public favors the option of physician-assisted suicide. Recent surveys of American physicians in Oregon and Michigan show that many doctors favor it too, as long as there is legal protection.

Discussions of assisted suicide are among the most personal conversations. They test our individual understanding of compassion, ethics and moral responsibility. Ethical issues raised by physician-assisted suicide cover the 20th century waterfront, from the right to die and proxy decision-making to physician professionalism and access to treatment.

How does managed care affect these four issues?

Right to die

Within managed care organizations, every member has a right to the organization's services. Should managed home care include assisted suicide services or should they be part of "demand management?" Should hospice care be part of those managed care services, and should seminars on pain management become a continuing medical education requirement? Should Dr. Kevorkian's little plastic clip become durable medical equipment? Should health systems consider outsourcing this particular assessment, or will they have the expertise to develop their own programs?

These questions about rights to treatment are perverse, but rights are interpreted as legal matters in our society, and conjure up thoughts of demands and suits.

Many medical ethical issues present as disagreement, and "rights" are sometimes invoked to settle them. Medical ethicists have often emphasized consensus-building—not "fighting for what's right"—as a way to solve clinical problems.

Medical ethicists have also taught that there is no legal right to die. Now, we're not so sure. The Second and Ninth Circuit Courts, within just a few weeks of one another, suggested that there is a constitutionally protected right to die.

This newly interpreted right to die is paradoxical, at best. There is no "right" to treatment in the United States, except in Veterans Administration hospitals, federal prisons, hospital emergency departments and managed care organizations.

Especially in managed care, we seem more interested in making sure patients don't get treatment they don't want than in assuring they get treatment they need—whether conventional, alternative or experimental. Perhaps the right-to-die movement can show the managed care community that this understanding is backwards.

Proxy decision-making

The federal Patient Self-Determination Act (PSDA) of 1990 requires that HMOs and hospitals, among others, ask whether a patient has an advance directive. A 1998 bill may extend the PSDA. Is there a designated decision-maker in case of an incapacitated patient? Such a decision-maker, 1990s reasoning goes, ought to represent what the patient wants, not what the proxy or family wants.

Data from the Netherlands indicate that physician-assisted suicide and euthanasia are disturbingly common among patients whose proxies request it for them. Holland is economically and socially homogenous when compared with the United States, and the financial pressures that managed care highlights here are nearly absent there.

If we lived in a culture in which family-centered decision-making were well accepted, American physicians might accept proxy requests for assisted suicide as equivalent to the patient request. Yet in our current logical, dichotomous way of thinking about right and wrong, such proxy, perhaps family-oriented requests seem inappropriate, and the violation of patient automony seems blatant.

If the Dutch experience of proxy decision-making for assisted suicide and euthanasia translates at all, the principles of population-based health and fairness to others have a long way to go for acceptance in managed care.

Professionalism

Professionalism is a do-or-die issue for physicians. Honest, well-meaning physicians disagree on whether we should help patients die. Some, like Timothy Quill, have become strong advocates for this view; others, like Edmund Pellegrino, have always been rigorously opposed.

There are arguments both ways. On the one hand, physicians should make it possible for their patients to take their own lives in exceptional circumstances with specific, triple-checked, publicly known criteria. On the other hand, **a patient's request for assisted suicide is often a symptom of the problem (from clinical depression to substandard palliative care) rather than a solution.**

Whatever we might think about assisted suicide, managed care counts on physician professionalism as much as or more than any other delivery system. A patient must be able to trust a doctor's judgment, derived from that patient's medical condition and personal circumstances. The financial incentives to physicians to limit care cannot be allowed to influence, much less distort our professional judgment, especially near the end of life.

Access to treatment

It is outrageous to posit access to a doctor's assistance in dying but not in living, especially for disadvantaged patients. Care for those who are living deserves the same protection as care for the dying, as they are equally important.

Managed care responds to a health care system that has previously paid for medically indigent care with cost-shifting from the rich to the poor. Even within a managed care organization, indigent patients are less able to pay for services and may not know how to argue for treatment to which they are entitled. It goes almost without saying that most such patients are women and minorities, some of whom had trouble gaining access to care in the first place.

The lowest-cost solution

Yes, there should be quality parameters and performance standards for gauging promptness and helpfulness in assessing and treating pain and suffering, for alleviating family burden, and for improving patient and family satisfaction with these tasks. But no, assisted suicide in managed care is not the answer. It is, however, the lowest-cost solution to nearly any patient problem. Separating ethics and economics is the least we can do.

For Further Reading:

1. Callahan S. A feminist case against euthanasia. Health Progress 1996; 77(6):21–29.
2. Emanuel EJ, Fairclough DL, Daniels ER, Clarridge BR. Euthanasia and physician assisted suicide: attitudes and experiences of oncology patients, oncologists and the public. Lancet 1996; 347:1805–1810.
3. Pellegrino ED. Beneficent killing: the false promise of euthanasia and assisted suicide. In Emanuel LL (ed). Physician Assisted Suicide and Euthanasia, Harvard University Press, Cambridge, 1998, in press.

2 3

Physician-Assisted Suicide and Managed Care: A Match Made in Hell

T HE U.S. S UPREME C OURT has decided that laws in New York and Washington states outlawing suicide were valid: **Physician-assisted suicide is not a constitutional right.**

The fact that so many patients—almost two-thirds in most polls—consistently seem to want a suicide option represents an opportunity for managed care to take the high road.

Not that it can afford to take any other. As Ren Mattlin of Los Angeles asked in a letter to *The New York Times* just before the Supreme Court's June 26 decision: "Why are we rushing to legalize assisted suicide before making every effort to get those of us living on the fringes to feel valued, or at least comfortable? I fear it is because, in this age of managed care, assisted suicide is cheaper."

Like Dennis Rodman, managed care has an image problem, at minimum. Even if physician-assisted suicide were both legally permissible and morally defensible as public policy, it would be the wrong thing for managed care. Why? No one would believe that managed care organizations really wanted to do the right thing. Everyone would think they wanted to do what would not cost much, and what would help them compete in the market.

Unlike Dennis Rodman, managed care cares deeply about

how much it gets paid. It is not in the game for love. And that's the problem.

Managed care must have a stronger sense of public mission than merely "the cheapest available option." It must strive to be the Gap, the Motorola, the Neiman-Marcus of health care systems, not the Dollar Store. Its service must be first-rate, and its concern about costs must be invisible behind its love of quality.

Facing patient's fears

Professionals working in managed care settings must explicitly address the fears of patients who request physician-assisted suicide. *Fear of suffocation. Fear of pain. Fear of suffering. Fear of being a burden.*

Nearly every physician has heard a patient say, "Doc, can't you give me something to, you know, take care of this if I can't go on?"

The ethical answer depends on whether you are a doctor to this patient.

Suicide is considered morally acceptable by some. But it is not *medically* **acceptable.** Sometimes, there seem to be good reasons for a person to feel life is not worth living, though such reasons can be reliably invoked only by a patient with full decision-making capacity. Profoundly disturbing studies in Australia and the Netherlands indicate that some patients' families and physicians are good—too good—at creating these reasons when the patients themselves do not.

But the personal moral act of assisting in a patient's suicide should not be dressed up in physician's clothing and called "medical." What medical justification could there be to kill a patient? It would be pretense to say that overprescribing narcotics or injecting potassium chloride or other such gruesome acts are "treatments." What is their indication? Contraindication? Adverse effects?

Can anyone, even experienced physicians, say that certain people are high enough on a miserableness scale that it is "rational" and "appropriate" to help them die? How far away from those clinical determinations is "medically necessary?" How can we compare these "worthy" patients with those whose illness is less advanced but whose spiritual sense of suffering is greater, or who have fewer family members to express their wishes?

The whole physician-assisted suicide business reeks. *It is the wrong business for managed care, already suspect for judgments about ethics and necessity.*

Better options

Attention to patient and family psychological, social and spiritual needs might be offered by a special quality-of-life team. Nonmedical needs are as important as medical ones, and they exist even for those dying patients who do not wish to refuse all life-sustaining measures. These patients too must be given the choice, comfort and dignity that ought to characterize care near the end of life.

If monitoring the quality of life at the end of life were part of the Health Plan Employer Data and Information Set (HEDIS) measurements, along with vaccination and pneumovax rates, then perhaps the demand for physician-assisted suicide would lessen.

If coding and registering "do not resuscitate" orders were routine and centralized, then emergency treatment and unwanted transfer to emergency departments from home and long-term care facilities might be prevented. More than half of the states now authorize nonhospital "do not resuscitate" forms, but none save Oregon authorize physician-assisted suicide.

These innovative approaches and others must be tested, evaluated, and—if patients find them helpful—implemented. As Christine Cassel, MD, and Bruce Vladeck, PhD, wrote in *The New England Journal of Medicine* in praise of a new diagnosis code for palliative care:

"It is never too late to provide greater comfort, especially since we have extraordinary pharmacologic and other tools with which to do so. Nothing is more gratifying than being able to relieve pain and suffering. Such gratification ought to be taught and modeled as one of the supreme satisfactions and rewards of the healing professions."

Because of managed care's potential for population-based

health, it can instill confidence and alleviate fear with more than one patient at a time.

An array of options exist for managed care organizations, including:

1. **Physician, physician assistant and nursing training in supportive care methods, skills and techniques;**
2. **Better physician knowledge about pain control;**
3. **Personal, focused advance care planning, with or without recorded advance directives** (which are often uninterpretable and seldom discussed with physician and proxy);
4. **Expanded use of hospice care,** and an expanded definition and scope of hospice itself; and
5. **Better communication about patients' fears of being a burden, of suffocating, of having pain, and of suffering.**

These goals may be hard for managed care to publicize or to feature on national billboards. But they are benefits that get back to people and their families and co-workers. Achieving these goals will help employers retain enrollees for the long term, especially in Medicare managed care. People remember who treated them well when Aunt Mary died.

And these changes can be embraced without the need for physician-assisted suicide.

For Further Reading:

1. Angell M. The Supreme Court and physician-assisted suicide—the ultimate right. New England Journal of Medicine 1997; 336:50–53.
2. Lynn J, Cohn F, Pickering JH, et al. The American Geriatrics Society on physician-assisted suicide: brief to the U.S. Supreme Court. Journal of the American Geriatrics Society 1997; 45:489–499.
3. Sulmasy DP. Managed care and managed death. Archives of Internal Medicine 1995; 155:133–135.

2 4

Advance Directives
in Managed Care:
Inspired by Love or Money?

ADVANCE DIRECTIVES are among the most studied topics in medical ethics. They are a logical approach to an intimate subject. Nearly everyone recommends them, but relatively few patients—a maximum of 25 percent, and probably fewer—have them.

Advance directives are controversial, and probably will become more so. There is keen interest in whether advance directives save money, can save money, and should be used to save money. The federal Patient Self-Determination Act (PSDA) requires managed care plans, among others, to educate their communities and to inform patients upon enrollment of their right to have an advance directive and to refuse treatment.

The basic facts

Written advance directives (living wills and durable power-of-attorney documents) are designed to allow people to determine how treatment decisions should be made when they themselves are unable to participate. Richard Nixon and Jacqueline Kennedy Onassis both completed living wills.

Almost all data about advance directives come from middle-class, educated Caucasian research subjects. But many new entrants to managed care are African-American, Hispanic and Asian. Denied access to much health care in the past, these groups have shown less interest in advance directives than Caucasian patients. Many American Indians, especially the Navajos, believe the whole idea is a curse.

People most likely to have advance directives are white, better educated and of higher socioeconomic class than average. Patients with some terminal illnesses, especially AIDS and cancer, have advance directives more often than others with equally grim prognoses—end-stage heart, liver and respiratory failure. Many people complete written advance directives on their own or on advice from legal counsel, without a clinician.

Chances are three out of four that if a hospitalized patient has an advance directive, hospital clinicians will not know about it.

Relatively few directives currently make it to the medical record. In one reported case ("The Bookie, the Girlfriend and the Vultures," *Annals of Internal Medicine* 1991; 114:98) a woman duped her groggy boyfriend into signing a limiting advance directive one morning and pulled the document (giving her decision-making control over his treatment) from her purse at the end of a long consultation with his doctor later that evening.

Several studies demonstrate that physicians are no better than chance at guessing their patients' preferences for life-sustaining treatment. Family members and proxies are only a little better than physicians. (For a detailed research review, see Miles, et al., "Advance End-of-Life Treatment Planning," *Archives of Internal Medicine* 1996; 156:1062–1068.)

Love

Advance directives were probably conceived as an act of love. The PSDA's intent was to allow patients to express their own values clearly and to encourage conversation among patients, family members and health professionals. Many patients who have completed advance directives allow their trusted proxy to override their expressed wishes. Patients more often intend their proxies to be designated hitters rather than messengers. Who makes decisions is as important as the content of the decision.

But advance planning (anticipatory discussions of decision-making capacity, realistic treatment goals and reasons) can reduce uncertainty. The process of understanding a patient's values, given his or her particular condition, is as important as a specific event such as intubation or hospice referral.

Some patient advocates, including many physicians, think there are better ways to show love than to complete a written advance directive. No 8.5" × 14" small-print form document captures the spirit of any person. Sometimes, for example, family unity may be the patient's most important value. Yet our autonomy-centered system does not accommodate working for the family (or the community) as easily as working for an individual.

Money

At least four peer-reviewed studies have been published about advance directives and saving money. The data are mixed and inconclusive. Not what you expected?

Fewer hospital ventilator purchases and positron emission tomography scans should mean lower costs if advance directives are used to limit unwanted treatment. Yet limiting treatment in the hospital means increasing its use elsewhere—at home, in a hospice or perhaps in a distant long-term care facility.

Advance directives were probably not generated to save money. The PSDA was part of a federal budget bill, however, and this fact influenced some of the current, accelerating concern about advance directives as cost-containment tools.

On a micro level, clinical assessments of proxy intent and reliability seldom reveal distorted judgment stemming from financial conflicts of interest between proxy and patient. But if foul play is suspected, physicians should report it to hospital management. On a macro level, economic opportunism calls loudly to those in the business of creating economic opportunities.

The real danger of advance directives in managed care is that they will be used to limit needed, useful, expensive

treatment under the guise of ethics. In a system that prizes cost containment, quality and, increasingly, service beyond nearly all else, this treachery can subvert even the best intentions.

To ensure their successful and ethical use, advance directives must be:

- understood as a signal for outpatient discussion of reasons for preferences;
- discussed with patient and proxy, together, in the same office visit;
- reviewed in the office, with a family visit reflecting the complex decision-making this review represents;
- interpreted in light of a patient's current decision-making capacity, and, if impaired, potential for recovering that capacity;
- seen as a major part of a managed care organization's community educational effort, focused on understanding patient values.

In the office, physicians should initiate routine discussions of advance planning as part of an annual history and physical, or health promotion/disease prevention assessment. In the hospital, the person asking about patient preferences should not be part of quality improvement, utilization review or risk management, and should speak with the patient directly.

Advance directives in managed care should be part of community service and demand management. They should be as tangible as educational videotapes and faxback technology for patients. They should mean role playing, continuing medical education courses, and advance planning office worksheets for physicians, physician assistants and nurses. And when brought to the office, they should be recognized as the red flags they are. The patient is saying: "Talk with me about this."

For Further Reading:

1. Emanuel LL. Structured advance planning: is it finally time for physician action and reimbursement? Journal of the American Medical Association 1995; 274:501-503.

2. Levinsky N. The purpose of advance medical planning—autonomy for patients or limitation of care? New England Journal of Medicine 1996; 335 (10):741–45.

3. Miles SH. Advance end-of-life treatment planning: A research review. Archives of Internal Medicine 1996; 156:1062–1068.

2 5

High-Tech Home Care

A colleague in a Southern state writes:

"A 35-year-old woman is paralyzed from C3 [the third cervical vertebra] down, secondary to a CVA [cerebrovascular accident, or stroke], and has a tracheostomy and a portable ventilator. The HMO says that she is 'custodial care' (not a covered benefit), wants to delegate the trach care to nurses' aides and eliminate home health service. The service, however, has refused, citing a Board of Nurse Examiners ruling that a licensed nurse could not delegate his/her duties to an unlicensed person.

"The HMO now wants to train neighbors and the patient's 10-year-old daughter to do the trach care. The patient's husband is a full-time state employee willing to quit his career to care for his wife."

THIS TRAGIC, MORALLY OUTRAGEOUS CASE demonstrates many of the ethical dilemmas in high-tech home care. Most of us who watched the Academy Awards saw Christopher Reeve, a C-2 ventilator-dependent quadriplegic, thank his community in measured breaths after his own terrible accident. Fewer of us caught the *New York Times* report of Reeve's third-party payer trouble, much the same as our patient's, resolved before that news report.

As with inpatient ethics, the issues can be sounded out using the framework spelled out in Jonsen, Siegler and Winslade's *Clinical Medical Ethics* [New York: McGraw-Hill, 4th edition, 1997]: medical indications, patient preferences, quality-of-life and contextual factors.

A supplement to the *Hastings Center Report* ["The Technological Tether," 1994; 24(5):51–528] helpfully clarifies the theory of high-tech home care ethics.

Medical indications

Good ethics needs sound facts. What is the patient's underlying illness, prognosis for recovery from the C3 event, and prognosis for vent independence? Over what time line? Is the primary goal to extend life, or palliate, or restore health? Are there other treatment protocols available in regional centers?

These are basic questions regarding what is medically possible. They are questions about whether this state is endless, or whether there is an achievable goal in sight, within an understood time period.

There are also technical medical questions about competent treatment administration. Unlikely to be technically difficult, for example, home trach care is still a skilled service, with contextual benefits and burdens not yet articulated.

Patient preferences

If the patient's capacity is present, issues of advance care planning—assigning authority to make decisions if she becomes incapacitated and discussing preferences about life-saving interventions—must be the second item (after goal-setting, above) on the agenda.

If the patient's decision-making capacity is impaired and cannot be improved, then obtaining a legal guardian is next. Guardianship is a legal procedure (probably needed to protect this patient from undertreatment, and the husband is a prime candidate for this post). **Documentation and discussion of the guardian's preferences, complemented by what is medically possible, is** *essential.*

Quality-of-life factors

Early patients on portable respirators called themselves "respinauts," raising interesting questions of identity. Is the respirator part of her? Or is she now part machine, forever tethered? Can she adjust her expectations of what life could be like in (presumably) endless quadriplegia? What would make life worth living, and is it achievable? If not, what is?

Most of us regard our homes as private, personal spaces, not mini-ICUs. **In high-tech home care, a home can lose a great deal of its warmth for healthy family members. Sometimes an intermediate institution can minimize the intrusions on privacy and disruptions of family life and maximize the use of limited financial resources.** And institutional treatment can provide psychological security for patient and caregiver which no home environment can match.

Contextual factors

What does a particular HMO contract actually say about home health? Does it have a limit on days or dollars? Even if it does, the HMO's obligation is not simply contractual. A contract, like law, is the *least* we have to do.

Is the patient's primary physician willing to call and write the medical director of the HMO and, with the director if possible and necessary, speak with the HMO CEO or Board? Should the home care nurse help set goals and advocate here too, as home care nurses are especially knowledgable about and close to the action?

Difficult questions of HMO resource allocation and policy are not answerable with this case. Home care expenses can easily be enormous and vary widely from vendor to vendor. Some physicians are routinely presented with care plans and equipment orders they haven't authorized but are asked to sign. If respirator services are carved out of the contract, should our dependent patient just go broke, go on television or die without them?

Public outrage with such cases has already reached *Newsweek* and ABC-TV's "20/20." **Limiting services when such obvious need exists reflects poorly on managed care as a whole, and on individual systems in particular.** Poor service comes back to bite such systems in advanced markets.

The family's burden in high-tech home care is daunting and unfair. The real difficulty in training home caregivers is the emotional impact of such treatment on them, the family and its life. Is there a moral obligation for a husband to give up his job—and likely, his health insurance—so that he can care for his wife? Or is there an obligation to support her in whatever way he is able, while keeping some of his life, and her health coverage support?

Finally, the Family and Medical Leave Act now provides limited job protection for the husband, but the leave is unpaid and brief. Of course, there is no school leave for the patient's daughter. "What if I do something wrong while suctioning Mommy?" is an especially horrific yoke to place on 10-year-old shoulders.

The tragedy of medicine is that illness happens, and the magic is that people somehow cope. What this patient and her family don't need is a cold financial shoulder without explicit attention to the ethical issues in the case. They do need:

- **Fact discovery and clarification, including prognosis and managed care terms;**
- A list of achievable medical and personal goals and a timeline and strategy for each;
- Consideration of legal guardianship;
- Advance care planning; and
- A search for alternative sources of home caregiving, including church and community members.

For Further Reading:

1. Fishman P, Von Korff M, Lozano P, Hecht J. Chronic care costs in managed care. Health Affairs 1997; 16(3):239–247.
2. Managing Medicare home care. Public Sector Contracting Report 1996; 2(11):171–172.
3. The technological tether. Hastings Center Report 1994; 24(5):S1–S28.

PART III

2 6

Respect and Communication Skills

Mr. Henderson is 72. He is worried about his prostate. His biopsy came back borderline, and his wife wants him to have an operation instead of an MRI and regular laboratory testing. Mr. Henderson has been married for 51 years, and he and his wife are in Dr. Beale's office.

"I don't know, Doc. Maybe I should have the surgery. We haven't had relations in two years—"

"Honey, you have cancer!" she says.

"But it isn't for sure, is it Doc?"

"Well, no."

"Your brother just died of cancer!" she says.

"Isn't there a pill I could take, Doc? Couldn't we just wait?"

"The kind of cancer the prostate may have," Dr. Beale says, "sometimes stays exactly where it is for five or ten years. About four times out of ten, men can't have full erections after an operation."

Mrs. Henderson bites her lip. "We're old, Doc, it doesn't matter," she says.

"Doc, how about that blood test now," Mr. Henderson says.

OW HAS RESPECT **for person changed in this era of managed care?** Has it grown, becoming more accepting, tolerant, personal and compassionate? Or has it dwindled, becoming more narrow-minded, indifferent, vague and stingy?

Before managed care, respect for persons had limited standing as an ethical principle. Patients asked that end-of-life care include excellent palliation as a first priority, and some physicians learned it. Families asked that patients unable to make decisions but without hope of recovery be allowed to die, and some more physicians allowed it. Women asked whether modified radical mastectomies and repeat Cesarean sections were really necessary, and many physicians found that they were not. Men asked why impotence had to accompany surgical treatment of benign prostatic hyperplasia if it was benign, and many, many physicians began to recommend watchful waiting.

In managed care, respect for persons has helped *populations* of patients, but has been less helpful to *individual* patients. On the one hand, pain relief and care near the end of life are near the top of the national ethics agenda. Mastectomy, Cesarean section, and transurethral resection of the prostate rates are all down; survival rates are stable; quality of life is up.

On the other hand, **there is less time than ever for developing sound doctor-patient relationships.** Doctor-patient-payer relationships seem to be more important than doctor-patient relationship to patients and payers. Individual physicians' practice patterns are being scrutinized for aberrancies. Homogeneity, conformance and quantifiable productivity are good; deviations from the mean are not. **Patients will switch physicians for a few dollars a month, and those few dollars seem to represent the value of the relationship.**

Culturally diverse care makes individual relationships even more tricky and time-intensive. Nonwhites entering managed care are disproportionately and expensively ill and have different understandings of patient preference, doing good, organizational obligation, fairness and relationship than do Caucasians.

Community by community, plans that can should suggest, initiate and emulate successful programs for integrating standardized recognition of nonCaucasian value systems into medical practice.

Here, there is also the potential for gaining the trust of people who have little reason to trust a health care system that does not provide health care for everyone, and from which they have been excluded until recently.

Physicians themselves also deserve respect. They have had little from managed care plans, payers and employers. Too many still feel disheartened and impotent. With the patient, they've noticed the 800-pound payer gorilla in the examining room, sometimes standing between the patient and a particular treatment. Do they game the system to gain access for that patient, and perhaps restore the patient's trust? Do they lie to account for the extra time and effort they spend daily, knowing that managed care often pursues short-term profits at the expense of long-term health?

Physicians don't do either. They don't lie for individuals or for themselves. Physicians should play by the rules—rules are part of life, and physicians should play square.

But physicians should try to change the rules when they are unfair and should try to regain some control over the direction of patient treatment. Patients want this, badly. Physicians should start by being focused: doing something very well clinically, educationally or administratively; being very clear about its documentation; managing its financial and personal risk well.

How can physicians give patients and themselves a little more control?

To patients who are basically well, physicians and managed care could offer incentives to achieve their clinical goals. Aligning incentives could work for well members—for example, Medicare members to date have been the "well elderly."

But it is not just the well elderly who will sign up for Medicare risk plans. The number of patients enrolled in Medicare managed care is expected to double to nearly 10 million by 2001. Medicare recipients are already swapping the price of their prescriptions for the identity of their physician.

Even more than younger patients, Medicare patients who are underdiagnosed or undertreated see these sins of omission as sins of commission. Incentives may mean little to them, and may even be twisted to discriminate especially against women, as most elderly people are women. There are no easy answers here.

Similarly, identifying the right business thing to do is not as easy as it may seem, but more important than ever. Tickets to see the Bulls, courtesy of industry representative X, and a tee time courtesy of industry representative Y are both kickbacks. These are surely not new practices, though just as surely they do not show respect for patients who ultimately pay for physician perks.

There are other small daily tradeoffs, and they are traded off differently by different physicians. A physician's need to hit cost-effectiveness targets may not lead to a 65-year-old woman's screening bone densitometry, still uncertain in value. Injectable calcitonin that comes out of the primary physician's cap may mean a referral to the rheumatologist to make the diagnosis of osteoporosis definitive and prescribe the ($1,400 monthly) medication. The estimated 60-minute visit needed to understand a Medicare patient's past six hospitalizations may mean seeing her three times for 20 minutes over three weeks, and seeing two other patients waiting to be seen, in rooms, now.

Whether these tradeoffs will increase the likelihood of malpractice liability suits is still uncertain. On the one hand, limiting patient choice of physicians and hospitals, and delaying referrals and authorizations cannot improve communication, respect and trust. On the other hand, first dollar coverage of bills, formal appeal and grievance procedures, patient representatives, internal quality improvement programs, financial incentives to reduce unnecessary or inappropriate care, and case management programs for high-risk patients probably *decrease* the likelihood of suit.

Reducing the malpractice risk

What are some practical rules for avoiding malpractice in managed care? The rules are much the same as in service-oriented indemnity medicine: communicate well, docu-

ment, believe in the goodness of a medical calling, don't succumb to the lure of easy money.

Never, ever change a patient's medical record except by lining through an entry, initialing and dating it. Spectrographic analysis catches even erased entries; Xerox copies of medical records are everywhere.

Call patients when they miss an appointment, and document the call. Write what patients say in quotes, and be prepared to let them read what you've written. Try to dictate or use a computer to enter notes—if you're not yet computer savvy, find a hospital or health system course and take one—even for three hours once. The payback will be enormous in legibility, speed and clarity.

Information is power. Here is some. The median malpractice payment since 1990 is $52,250, and the average payment is $154,404; in 1996, it was $75,000 and $183,126. More malpractice payments than any year previously—19,927—were made in 1996.

HMOs made almost 40 percent of the 2.76 million queries to the Data Bank in 1996—far more than did mandated organizations such as hospitals and licensing boards. The Data Bank received a record number of reportable actions in 1996, and more than 80 percent of these were licensure actions. Hospital clinical privilege reports to the Data Bank are expected to increase in coming years.

Physicians and practice managers who learn basic principles of ethics will improve their decision-making and have to spend less time covering colleagues who are occupied by the drudgery and anxiety of malpractice suits.

Solving ethical problems before they become legal ones should be a first step for physicians who practice in managed care. Prior to managed care, writing appropriate do-not-resuscitate orders and assuring and documenting informed consent to surgical procedures were ways to prevent legal problems. Researching whether a specific treatment is experimental, deciding what services are owed to surrounding geographic communities, and deciding which billing, coding and referring practices are acceptable and which are not are newer ways to use ethics to anticipate legal predicament.

Respect for persons in managed care: the road ahead

Respect for persons is critical to the success and survival of managed care. Although physicians as a group are often viewed as fallen angels, physicians as individuals still survive as honorable and even heroic. And after all is said and done, medicine is still practiced person-to-person.

Physicians who can understand more specifically what a patient wants, or what his family wants, will set the gold standard for communication. Discovering why patients want what they want is as important as what they want. Giving patients the opportunity to explain their values is keenly important and means their patronage.

Patients want to forgive physicians for not learning palliative care quickly enough and for performing unnecessary procedures. Patients still want a personal relationship, and they will get as much of one as doctors can give. What patients will give up is much of the relationship's continuity, which many will accept as worth trading for its reduced cost.

What can clinicians do to respect patients as persons and to create satisfactory relationships with them?

1. **Orient patients to the process of the visit when they first come in.** Say "First, I'll examine you and then we'll talk the problem over" or "I will leave time for your questions."
2. **Pick up on new health care language,** and listen for new names and titles for old positions and roles, without scoffing. Some physicians hate being called "providers"; many patients don't mind at all being called "customers." Surely physicians and providers can help patients and customers feel important, appreciated and well served.
3. **Laugh more with patients.** Laughing shows that you enjoy

them, that you enjoy humor, that you can be warm and empathetic and friendly. Friendliness with patients does not
cross any professional boundaries that should never be
crossed, and it helps to connect patients and physicians as
people, instead of as diseases and disease-fighters.

4. **Try not to make patients feel rushed or ignored.** If
there is no time to give an adequate explanation of the problem or treatment, have a team member schedule another appointment within a week for the patient before he or she
leaves.

5. **Break bad news and inform patients about mistakes
judiciously, kindly, directly and with hope for the future. Schedule extra time for such a patient,** at either
end of the day, when possible.

6. **Give more information about lifestyle and the psychosocial aspects of care.** People want information as
much as or more than they want to make decisions.

7. **Offer your patients your e-mail address.** As more people get on the Internet, physicians will be able to avoid
phone tag, phrase replies carefully and with subtlety, and give
patients the opportunity to write things they cannot bring
themselves to say.

8. **Try an A B C D E with difficult patients, who may be
demanding, frightened, angry, misinformed or all of
these.**

9. Admit there is a problem. Many patients will be relieved by
this acknowledgement.

10. Be kind and compassionate: People need to know that their
time is as or more valuable than their clinicians' and that they
deserve empathy or sympathy.

11. Create a context for meaning: The urgently evaluated skin
lesion may be just an ordinary nevus to a clinician but a
melanoma-in-situ to the 30-year-old whose mother has a
new diagnosis of colon cancer.

12. Draw some lines—boundaries to professional interactions

include time available, language acceptable, and topics for discussion.

13. Engage other sources for help—home health agencies, community and church groups, Internet information sites, and hospital-based wellness groups.

27

Does the Doctor-Patient Relationship Mean More to Doctors than to Patients?

THE DOCTOR-PATIENT RELATIONSHIP is the foundation of modern medical ethics. It is the touchstone for professional conduct and the single matter that physicians, when polled, say they value most about medical practice. But the doctor-patient relationship is changing, and so are medical ethics. To maintain the values that doctors and patients appreciate most, the profession may need another credible touchstone.

While principles of medical ethics are essentially the same for physicians working in fee-for-service practice as they are for those in capitated managed care, managed care does highlight certain serious concerns. Five important questions are:

- **How much coverage is fair**—to individuals, and to communities?
- **Who should control disclosure of financial conflicts of interest,** which ones and when?
- **Is lying to ensure a patient receives coverage ever right?**
- **What treatments are "marginal," "futile," and "experimental"**—and who should pay for them?

• Should private companies support public trusts, such as research, teaching and care of the indigent?

Lurking behind each question is the disturbing body of evidence that the doctor-patient relationship is more important to doctors than to patients. The kind of relationship most physicians were weaned on was covenantal, continuous, confidential, supportive and personal. But is it still?

Covenant or contract?

Fidelity and altruism are supposed to govern the doctor-patient relationship. Professionals put their patients' interests before their own, and pledge to defend those interests against administrative, medical and personal barriers. Yet more patients and doctors meet each other while under contract than ever before, and usually neither has truly free choice in the matter. In fact, patients as a whole are increasingly wary of physicians as a group, and think that physicians are paid too much—even while underestimating their income by half. At least one court has ruled that the doctor-patient relationship begins when the patient selects a primary care physician from a list.

Continuous or episodic?

A few years ago, I was privileged to practice with a partner who had taken care of three generations of the same family—of several families, in fact. Such continuity still exists, but it is rare as physicians couple and uncouple in group arrangements and are selected and deselected by managed care plans.

There is other evidence of indifference to the long-term promise of the doctor-patient relationship. Mall medical offices and urgent care centers sometimes pick up what slips through the cracks inside of hospitals and clinics. Separate inpatient and outpatient physicians and practices grow rapidly. Specialists must either build niche practices, teach generalists or retrain as generalists themselves. Few

endocrinologists are able to continue their long-term relationships with their diabetics, for example.

Patients increasingly regard the doctor-patient relationship as ripe for a no-fault divorce, and at least one study has shown that a difference of $20 per month is enough to separate one from one's doctor. A study done by the Commonwealth Fund in Boston, Los Angeles and Miami showed that 41 percent of managed care patients surveyed had changed doctors at least once in the past three years. Nowadays, the most common reason for a new patient visit to my office is "change of insurance."

Confidential or wide open?

The obligation to keep to oneself all information learned from or about the patient was called a "decrepit concept" 20 years ago in a seminal *New England Journal of Medicine* article. Mark Siegler determined that **more than 70 physicians, nurses, trainees, students and managers had access to a hospitalized patient's chart. Today, that number can be multiplied by three orders of magnitude.** As information systems record and beam bits of data we thought we'd told no one else to a cyberspace too big to think about, confidentiality of medical records seems like food for earthworms.

There's a well-known flip side to truthtelling here. It's "gag rules"—prohibitions on doctors' discussions with patients about how their insurance works, and what financial arrangements physicians have with payers. Yet the simple truth is that cost and information about it matter to patients—as much as or more than our own measures of satisfaction and service.

Collegial or solitary?

Advocacy is the first rule of traditional medical ethics. Trying to define the patient's disease process, eradicating the smallest discomforting lesion, gaining the wisdom of another colleague—all of these goals have motivated

referrals. Happily for physicians, the scientific philosophy implied by these goals has also been financially rewarding.

Yet in managed care, the financial incentives are reversed, and physicians face disincentives to refer, and to prescribe an off-formulary medication. To minimize the distortion of physician judgment, proposed rules from the Health Care Financing Administration limit the amount of compensation physicians can risk.

Personal or population-based?

Medical practice is nothing if not personal. Patients in the waiting room do not think of unidentifiable others when they are in the exam room, cold and naked but for a paper gown, waiting to be seen. Perhaps they should; perhaps we should all have a better, stronger, more global sense of community in this age of the Internet. But many of my patients find it hard enough to survive themselves without worrying about the world.

Managed care's ethical foundation is population-based. It is the health of the public that matters (including the public that is locked out)—even out of managed care. Rates of Pap smears, mammography and asthmatic hospitalization are criteria by which some health plans have already been judged by the National Committee for Quality Assurance. Infant mortality rates, overall length of hospital stay and the safety of new mothers discharged within 24 hours of birth are not far behind. Will medical responsibility for those persons who live within the managed care organization's shadow follow? Will practice guidelines that govern group practice let individual doctors and patients be personal?

Do other credible touchstones for modern medical ethics exist, now that the doctor-patient relationship isn't what it used to be? A moral relationship between payers and patients is one possibility; an integration of fairness to all with the choices of an individual is another. But for the time being, despite all the pressures upon it, the individual doctor-patient relationship is likely to remain the most important relationship in medicine—at least to doctors.

For Further Reading:

1. Emanuel EJ, Dubler NN. Preserving the physician-patient relationship in the era of managed care. Journal of the American Medical Association 1995; 273:323–329.
2. Mechanic D, Schlesinger M. The impact of managed care on patients' trust in medical care and their physicians. Journal of the American Medical Association 1996; 275:1693–1697.
3. Weiss LJ, Blustein J. Faithful patients: the effect of long-term physician-patient relationships on the costs and use of health care by older Americans. American Journal of Public Health 1996; 124:497–504; editorial 1699–1700.

2 8

How Much Should Doctors, Patients and Plans Care about Each Other?

H ERE IN CHICAGO, of the rugged elbows and tat-
tooed muscular shoulders that carry the Bulls, only basketball lets people believe we all live in the city that
works.

Basketball makes Bloomingdales shoppers and K-mart shoppers believe that they share the same values. Amazingly, basketball
creates a community.

Driving across Chicago this week, I noticed a billboard claim-
ing "We Hear You," next to a giant ear. Another billboard, with
a happy family as backdrop, announced "More Choices, Better
Value." A third had no graphics, just text: "We're Your Health
Plan, Not Your Doctor."

What sort of community makes it seem extraordinary that
doctors listen to patients? Why does one community health plan
promote choice for consumers, instead of unity and shared fortune
for citizens, as its value? Why does another plan separate "health"
and doctors? Are doctors, patients and health plans one community or three?

Physician community

Doctors behave as a group, and in many ways, we are not different from other groups. As workers, we do more of what we are paid well to do. As fraternity and sorority brothers and sisters, we try to take care of our own. As colleagues, we try to uphold professionalism. As leaders, we set the tone for our practices, and to some extent, our communities.

As a group, doctors are disappointed and bitter these days, though not so much about the way managed care has changed practice, reducing marginally effective care and futile care. The disappointment is not about shortened hospital stays or lengthened home health visits without commensurate charges.

Physicians' disappointment centers on overwhelming amounts of paperwork, "Big Brother" overseeing every move, and, in no small measure, the issue of money. Most doctors don't have the training to talk about money in a way that benefits our patients. The language of money in the clinic is unfamiliar to most doctors—sterile and corporate and without feeling, like the language of administration. Cost-effective treatment with a good loss ratio is one thing; defervescence after a four-day course of intravenous antibiotics, when your 65-year-old chronic lunger seemed destined for the intensive care unit, is quite another.

Some physicians are pessimistic about community and see our group split into winners and losers, or generalists and specialists. Other physicians want to remain optimistic and, though tired of red tape, onerous approval processes and the pressure to see more patients, have begun to innovate.

Some physicians have begun to unionize. Others have joined the ranks of physician executives and are trying to keep one foot in both camps. Still others have become entrepreneurs and developed ways to increase and promote satisfaction in their practices, transforming their own offices and clinics into communities unto themselves. Ever individuals, most physicians still have trouble thinking of themselves as having just one voice.

Patient community

Patients can also behave cohesively but, like doctors, don't think of themselves as members of a single group. As workers themselves, they try to make a living and hope their employers pay for insurance. As parents and children and spouses, they value their families and their families' health, sometimes before their own. As community members, they care about public health, especially as it affects them individually.

Individual patients are not disappointed with their individual physicians, but with physicians as a group. Physicians are thought to make too much money, spend too little time, run chronically late and have God complexes. Patients know physicians have financial conflicts of interest in managed care and are worried about them. Thankfully, patients have not yet held physicians responsible for "drive-by deliveries" or, more recently, fewer than four days' hospital stay post-mastectomy.

What do patients want? Well, from their own physicians, they want attention, trust, personal care and time. Evidence of compassion and excellent communication skills are also desirable. A neat appearance, promptness and ordinary courtesy also help.

Patients also want doctors to practice with cost in mind, but not first in mind. But why do patients as a whole want prudence? To know that resources are stewarded wisely, and being saved for those who really need them? Or to avoid being subjected to unnecessary procedures, and their potential financial, medical and personal cost?

If the former is true, then patients who signed up at work for Too Good HMO understand population-based health and principles on which good managed care is founded. Their assumption is that all Too Good HMO members are in it together. They are believers in public health, community and justice.

If the latter is true, then patients are watching out for themselves as individuals, and for their families. Their assumption often is that their monthly premium goes for their own health care—not someone else's. These are people just trying to make a living every day, and trying hard to make good choices.

Given patients who have diverse values and desires, is there a community in managed care? There *are* communities of covered lives, but HMO communities lack the shared assumptions and values characteristic of recognizable communities like school, work and home. Traditional communities have face-to-face contact. Members share at least one belief. They care for and even recognize each other. Many try to be fair and responsible.

Health plans recruit new members aggressively. Here in Chicago, there has not been the same effort to retain old ones, but in other parts of the country with greater managed care penetration, competition for retention is fierce. In Albuquerque, for example, plans advertise their mammography rates in hope of retaining their customers.

But for all the scoffing at managed care organizations, especially those whose sense of community seems tied to their stock price, these organizations can take moral positions currently out of reach of ordinary, individual doctors and patients. How? By deciding whom to contract with for services and whom to avoid serving.

Physicians, patients and executives could act as a population with shared values—as one community, instead of three. But to pull doctors, patients and health plans together, the shared values will have to be explicit, even if they turn out to be money, prudence and fairness to others.

For Further Reading:

1. Burzynski MA. Managed care: meeting employer, enrollee and community expectations. American Journal of Managed Care 1996; 2(6):707–710.
2. Jecker NS. Genetic testing and the social responsibility of private health insurance companies. Law, Medicine and Health Care 1992; 21(1):102–108.
3. Gray BH. Trust and trustworthy care in the managed care era. Health Affairs 1997; 16(1):34–49.

2 9

Managed Care "Menage à Trois": Doctor, Patient and Payer

THE RELATIONSHIP of doctor and patient is the foundation of modern medical ethics, and the roles of both doctor and patient are shifting. **Doctors and patients can expect at least three major changes in their relationship.** While physicians may not welcome these changes in every respect, they can anticipate them, prepare for them, and use them to prepare for the future. They are:

1. **A change in ethical principle. Justice, not autonomy, will be the most important principle.** Self-determination (autonomy) has operated independently of fairness to others (justice) in the choice and control-crazy late 20th century. But in managed care, there are plan members and community members other than the one who is ill then and there to worry about. An individual patient's best interests may have to be balanced against the interests of other patients because resources are limited.

   As a society, we are no longer content to have physicians order all possible tests and treatments for all patients in need, yet each individual patient still wants whatever tests and treatments he or she needs. And why not? Individuals seldom think of themselves as part of a managed care community of covered lives that pays individual bills. Such a community is hard for most patients to identify, much less identify with. Yet individuals are part of a community, and justice makes the community possible.

2. **A change in the players. The linear relationship of patient and physician is becoming a triangle: doctor, patient and payer. This is morally supportable if the payer can speak for the values of all patients and where they want their resources spent.**

Customers of managed care organizations have the opportunity to vote with their feet. If patients decide to favor technologies that value quality of life as much as survival, for example, more managed care resources could be directed to quality-of-life care. The hazard? The public may be unprepared to believe that managed care wants to excel at quality of life at the end of life, and may see it as a euphemism for saving money. And the real customers are employers—not patients.

3. **A change in service. Gatekeeping is a dirty word in managed care. Physicians can see their role more positively if they can define quality evaluation as a professional responsibility, or guide patients through the system to gain access to the care they need. Financial incentives to physicians to promote value, document outcomes, reduce costs and improve patient satisfaction will result in better, more service-oriented practice.**

Although the doctor-patient relationship will continue to change, physicians—especially generalists—can guide the direction of that change. **To really be successful, managed care plans and physicians must find a way to have rewarding, productive relationships—with each other and with patients.** Achieving this goal will require honesty and fidelity from all parties, virtues that the doctor-patient relationship has always required.

For Further Reading:

1. La Puma J. Anticipated changes in the doctor-patient relationship in the managed care and managed competition of the Health Security Act of 1993. Archives of Family Medicine 1994; 3:665–671.
2. Lipkin M. The corporatization of American medicine: the impact of managed care on the doctor-patient relationship. American Journal of Managed Care 1996; 2(6):734–737.
3. Sulmasy D. Physicians, cost control and ethics. Annals of Internal Medicine 1992; 116:920–926.

3 0

How and How Much Should Physicians Be Paid?

T HE OLDEST MEDICAL ETHICAL TENSION is one between a physician's inherent altruism and essential self-interest. But how much should a capitated managed care physician be paid?

The facts

Defined as a flat "fee per head per time," capitation is a way of sharing financial risk, something that many physicians now want to do. A plan's capitation rate may be adjusted for the age, gender, family size, demographics, projected medical costs and geographical characteristics of a patient population, and it ordinarily includes payment for certain services and excludes payment for others.

Other methods of compensation are also used in managed care—fee-for-service, discounted fee-for-service, relative value scale and straight salary. The results of patient satisfaction questionnaires about service (e.g., promptness, accessibility, sensitivity, communication skills) can modify a physician's compensation. So can utilization of labs, drugs and procedures. Bonuses and withholds may be tied

to individual volume targets and formulary compliance, or tied to targets for the medical group as a whole.

Physicians are already forced to balance the cost of their own compensation against the resources they authorize for patients and their health care. Like most other workers, physicians do more of what they are paid to do, and are influenced by financial incentives. Unlike most other workers, however—or at least to a greater degree—physicians have professional ethical obligations that influence compensation plans and terms.

The rules

In 1847, the AMA discussed issues of practice management and etiquette in its Code of Ethics. In 1995, the AMA's Council on Ethical and Judicial Affairs answered questions on the gatekeeper role and financial conflicts of interest in managed care.

In March 1996, the Department of Health and Human Services issued rules limiting physician rewards in Medicare and Medicaid managed care and mandating stop-loss insurance for a physician loss of more than 25 percent of overall compensation. The rules also require HMOs to disclose publicly their financial incentives to limit treatment and referrals.

For a while, the Clinton administration suspended enforcement of the rules, according to the July 8, 1996 *New York Times*, because HMOs objected to them. Medical professional groups had celebrated the rules as a clear message to the public that managed care doctors are not for sale. The reasoning: Patients who emerge from an annual exam without lab tests shouldn't have to wonder about their doctor's motivation. Was their doctor actually trying to hoard monies to pay for another HMO patient? Or was their doctor trying to earn a bonus?

What kind of incentives are ethical? Negative incentives to provide care that utilize general considerations of cost, benefit and effectiveness data can be appropriate. Yet such incentives should not be used as micromanagement tools that reduce care below prudent, empathetic levels. Positive financial incentives and risk reduction to provide care can

also be appropriate. **These incentives, however, carry the potential for iatrogenic injury, patient inconvenience and extra cost.**

What if we measured and rewarded quality care based on relieving the suffering of patients and the burdens on families? Or providing advance planning and improved aggressive care near death? Or maintaining functional status and patient and family satisfaction? Benchmarks of quality should be used as financial incentives to improve compensation, benefiting both patient and physician.

What kind of incentives are unethical? Negative incentives that simply save the employer or HMO money put the doctor and patient in adversarial positions. Financial conflicts of interests can easily become distorted clinical judgments—and one can slide into the other. Positive incentives that create patient-based revenue but do not benefit the health of patients are also unethical. Appointment cranking for monthly cholesterol levels or fully-billed daily blood-pressure checks are abusive.

Withholding money from a physician's capitation fee can pit physician against patient as do few other methods of payment, and do no one a favor. Too few physicians in too small a group caring for too few patients make balancing the mortgage versus ordering an MRI for a patient an impossible decision. Therefore, even while making it easier for physicians to make more money by suspending managed care regulation, the government just made it harder for managed care and managed care physicians to claim moral ground.

Are all doctors equal?

Medical practitioners have long been rewarded on the basis of their usefulness to the health of the community as a whole. Over at least eight centuries, physicians as a class have earned approximately four times the average societal wage, with many different societies' approval and endorsement.

Although all physicians have matriculated through generally

comparable curricula in generally comparable lengths of time, other important common values are different. Thus, physicians are not and should not be compensated equally in comparison with one another.

But what pay is fair for different individuals? Money alone? Nonmonetary forms of compensation should be considered as payment, such as time made available for personal and educational obligations, and for intellectual, emotional and humanistic challenge and fulfillment.

In physician payment, we must call upon a modern medical ethics that emphasizes fairness to patients as a whole and to physicians as a community. Physicians are not isolated, free agents who are justified in gaining for themselves whatever they can, without due regard for the interests of others in the community. We are members of a community of medical professionals and should be paid as members of that community.

Absent enforcement of the new Health and Human Services rules, an unregulated frontier of payment possibilities, has just been officially sanctioned. Many physicians would prepare themselves for some sacrifice as a profession on behalf of our patients as a whole if we were persuaded that greater access to care and investment in prevention and treatment would result. Yet few physicians are persuaded—a critical fact at a time when managed care's credibility is poor except as a system of cost constraint.

For Further Reading:

1. Billi JE, Wise CG, Bills EA, Mitchell RL. Potential effects of managed care on specialty practice at a university medical center. New England Journal of Medicine 1995; 333:979–983.
2. Kaplan SH, Greenfield S, Gandek B, Rogers WH, Ware JE, Jr. Characteristics of physicians with participatory decision-making styles. Annals of Internal Medicine 1996; 124:497–504.
3. Simon CJ, Born PH. Physician earnings in a changing managed care environment. Health Affairs 1996; 15(3):124–133.

3 1

Risk Management: Does Doing the Right Business Thing Decrease the Risk of Being Sued?

PHYSICIANS AND EXECUTIVES worried about liability are starting to pay some serious attention to ethics. **Physicians know that ethical breaches could cost them something more than patients and money: their reputations for professional integrity.**

Can lawsuits be avoided when there is barely office time to write out selective serotonin reuptake inhibitor (SSRI) prescriptions, much less discover that a patient's daughter was hospitalized last week for a drug overdose?

Doing the right thing was never so safe. *Or so necessary.*

Billing, coding and referring

Many systems push physicians to be worker bees and produce more for less. Rapid patient turnover has many forms, and one of them is "churning"—seeing patients weekly for blood pressure checks or monthly for cholesterol tests, for example. Medicare measures to reduce churning are weak and easily evaded.

"Churning" should have gone out with home butter production. Most physicians hate it, and it fits poorly with the way most are—entrepreneurial, achievement-oriented, independent.

It is one thing to hold seminars instructing physicians how to bill for procedures previously unrecognized as compensable (complex family meetings, for example). It is quite another to ignore or encourage systematic upcoding, unbundling of procedures or gaming the system to code what is not there. **Recording histories that were never taken or examinations that were never performed, and then billing for them, will destroy medicine as a profession.**

Subtle coding changes can become routine within a matter of weeks, and soon they don't seem like changes at all. Some British generalists have described dialysis to eligible 60-year-olds as "not indicated" when in truth it was not available because of systemwide allocation decisions. As economic forces have changed clinical judgment, so have they changed coding judgment.

Business judgment can also be distorted by the promise of easy money. Self-referral and kickbacks are not made any more beneficent because they are filtered through a hospital or hospital system. Physicians caught with their hand in the till are destined for the same kind of cell as the executives who hired them—or maybe one not quite as nice.

Referral has another dark side. It has been an ethical problem since the first time someone told a primary care physician that his or her patient could not see a specialist. Shortly thereafter, a specialist demonstrated that a primary care doctor had missed a melanoma, or had inefficiently managed a myocardial infarction, or had only three days' laparoscopy training before offering the procedure.

Issues of professionalism, competence, education, and promise-keeping are raised when a referral is denied or approved with conditions. Unknown specialists 26 miles from the patient's home or office are inconvenient and often transient, as whose turn it is to be credentialed seems to change annually. The inconvenience and confusion of obtaining a referral seems certain to frustrate, discourage and anger any middle-aged patient with nephrotic syndrome who, after all, wants only to know whether she really needs a kidney biopsy.

From student days onward, physicians probably learn best from each other, about particular cases, and in informal settings—the parking lot, the clinic hallway, the Internet chat room. Pushing doctors to spend less time learning about their patients can only make for reduced doctor-patient communication, greater feelings of inadequacy and vulnerability, and a void where professionalism should be.

Physicians change behavior in response to the law, and especially in response to malpractice suits. Harvard researcher Lucian Leape, M.D., and colleagues have documented that only 5 percent of significant inpatient errors are ever reported. Those reported are often linked to patient satisfaction and doctor-patient communication.

Unfortunately for physicians, the first things to go in shortened office visits are psychosocial interactions. **The core components of patient satisfaction—emotional support, attentiveness and partnership—are hard to provide in 10 minutes of face time.** Physicians who want to stay employed have heard the time-crunched message. Dissatisfaction and some patient turnover are now expected, but also unnecessary.

Johns Hopkins's Debra Roter and colleagues recently documented very high satisfaction with visits that just discussed problems of daily living, feelings and social relationships. Physicians liked these visits, and they also liked "consumerist" visits, in which they answered questions about patient health instead of asking them.

Contracts are the bane of many physicians' existence, because many were never trained to read them, or have been too naive to hire someone who can. No-appeal restrictive covenants, 30-day deselection and gag clauses are immoral facts of too many lives.

The doctor-patient relationship now usually depends on a payer for its existence, and the real payer is the employer. Health insurance is linked to employment, and job security is history. Presto chango: The doctor-patient covenant is now a contract, easily truncated by someone else's pen.

When Congress legislates how many days a patient should be hospitalized, or what disease du jour should receive special allowance, the quality of care goes down. Congress didn't go to medical school—most of it, anyway—and it has never seen a patient in the middle of the night or on Saturday afternoon. Doctors and patients, not legislators, should make therapeutic decisions.

Managed care could provide the very best for patients and tap creativity and compassion. It could reward patients who do more for themselves. It could find diabetics and hypertensives just as soon as they enroll, and prevent complications. It could use ethics committees to review policies before they are implemented. It could create a clinical consulting service for tough cases. It could recommend guidelines on limitation of marginal and futile treatment.

By marketing giant Porter Novelli's recent assessment, managed care companies are rated only slightly more believable than tobacco companies. **Tobacco's legal time has come: Managed care is next, unless it finds a way to support physicians who want to solve ethical problems before they become legal ones.**

Managed care has this chance, before its executives and even its physicians are sued for unethical business practices that have sullied managed care medicine's reputation and made it one of the least trusted industries in America. Toll-free corporate integrity programs designed to help comply with mandates and regulations offer a clean route to doing right, but few physicians have the time to call another 800 number while their patient waits.

For Further Reading:

1. Beckman HB, Markakis KM, Suchman AL, Frankel RM. The doctor-plaintiff relationship: lessons from plaintiff depositions. Archives of Internal Medicine 1994; 154:1365–1370.
2. Health Resources and Services Administration. 1996 Annual Report for the National Practitioner Data Bank. U.S. Department of Health and Human Services, Public Health Service, Health Resources and Services Administration, Bureau of Health Professions, Division of Quality Assurance, Rockville MD, 1997.
3. Levinson W. Physician-patient communication: a key to malpractice prevention. Journal of the American Medical Association 1994; 273:1619–1620.

3 2

Understanding and Protecting Medical Ethics Can Reduce Your Liability Risk

F EW PATIENTS acknowledge the inevitability of tragedy and suffering, and many hospital patients demand that someone in the institution restore them to wholeness. As medicine becomes more of a consumer good and less of a calling, physicians can call upon new colleagues—risk managers. The ethics of risk management requires a sense of balance and principle, as time and money spent upfront may pay dividends in quality care and patient satisfaction later.

Good risk management relies on a solid foundation in medical ethics. Skills risk managers use to reduce institutional liability parallel skills physicians use when resolving a clinical ethical dilemma. These include:

- **Identifying and clarifying the dilemma**
- **Demonstrating good judgment**
- **Communicating effectively**
- **Facilitating negotiation**
- **Constantly improving decision-making**

Using these skills can reduce a physician's and an institution's risk of liability exposure. Resolving conflicts of coverage, appealing financial limits on a patient's experimental treatment, and balancing corporate, personal and social accountability in a cost-constrained world are highlighted in managed care. Three cases illustrate these problems.

Case 1: Pre-admission testing and hospital policy

A 49-year-old woman with a cerebellar tumor comes to the hospital for a cerebral angiogram. The patient is waiting in the radiology department in a semi-sedated state after her angiogram. The hospital now refuses to admit her, as her HMO does not contract with it. A nearby facility is willing to admit her, but doesn't have a neurosurgeon on staff. The risk manager is called by the patient's primary care physician.

Pre-admission testing and post-procedure certification are the areas of managed care that physicians dislike most. If physicians appeal cases like this to risk managers, a bonus can result: Changes in institutional policy can follow from the particular case.

Policy making will be an area of excellence for the first-rate ethics committee of the managed care future. Both physicians and risk managers can assist ethics committees with policy formation, and help them implement and evaluate policies, particularly about institutional processes that do not facilitate care, but should.

Case 2: When experimental care is medically necessary

A 42-year-old business executive wants to try naltrexone for alcoholism, which is considered an innovative treatment—FDA-approved for one purpose, but prescribed for another. The patient has been admitted several times over the past several years, most recently with a serious alcohol withdrawal syndrome. The patient's attorney threatens the physician, the managed care organization and the hospital with lawsuit unless the patient receives naltrexone.

Innovative or experimental treatment is sometimes difficult to define, may be very expensive, and may increase patient, physician and manager expectations and frustrations. Risk managers and top management may be tempted to make general rules about all experimental treatments, but this is hazardous. Instead, each case and each treatment should be considered on its own merits, each time conflict arises.

Patients who use attorneys to make threats for them get more of what they want in managed care. Wanting and needing are different, however, and an innovative treatment is somewhere between research and therapy. Informed consent to research demands a higher standard—better information, greater understanding, complete volition—than informed consent to treatment. The patient should be prepared to help set the goals as if the in-between service were treatment and accept the risks as if it were research. Innovative treatment is, after all, unproven.

Case 3: Spending resources to save resources

At a time when the hospital's operating rooms are full and won't have an opening for two days, a young woman needs semi-emergent heart surgery. She is a 27-year-old heroin user and HMO member who needs a mitral valve replacement for endocarditis. She's been hospitalized two weeks for intravenous antibiotics and is no longer febrile, but her valve and cardiovascular condition have deteriorated. Utilization management has asked the primary care physician to discharge her until the operating room can take her.

Learning about proper documentation is the linchpin of liability prevention. Holding, recording and quoting meetings; titling, dating and timing notes; photocopying, carbon-copying and keeping notes about disagreements—are techniques that clinical ethics offers that enable physicians to reduce risk.

What would a physician skilled in ethics and risk management say about these cases?

For the 49-year-old post-angiogram patient, the cost of a 23-hour stay is very small compared with the potential negative public relations generated by the transfer of a groggy, invaded patient to a competitor.

162 MANAGED CARE ETHICS

For the 42-year-old alcoholic whose lawyer threatens a frivolous lawsuit, a time-limited trial of therapy would be reasonable, with a contractual agreement with the patient to discontinue the medication unless objective beneficial effects are seen at a follow-up visit.

For the 27-year-old heroin user whose mitral valve is greatly damaged, discharging her will enable her to use heroin more easily, further lengthening her next stay, and likely costing other HMO members more than the cost for two days' extra hospitalization.

Avoiding liability

Physicians who learn and master basic skills in clinical ethics can reduce their risk of getting entangled in major liability situations. This will also help meet tough new institutional requirements from the Joint Commission on Accreditation of Healthcare Organizations for accreditation in ethics.

Adapted and excerpted in part from La Puma J, Schiedermayer DL, "Ethics, Accreditation and Managed Care: A Guide for Risk Managers," in Youngberg B. (ed), Reducing the Emerging Risks of Managed Care, Aspen Publishers, Gaithersburg, Md., 1997.

For Further Reading:

1. Roter DL, Stewart M, Putnam SM, Lipkin M, Stiles W, Inui TS. Communication patterns of primary care physicians. Journal of the American Medical Association 1997; 277:350–356.
2. Gosfield AG. The legal subtext of the managed care environment: a practitioner's perspective. Journal of Law, Medicine and Ethics 1995; 23(3):230–235.
3. Levinson W, Roter D, Mullooly JP, Dull VT, Frankel RM. Physician-patient communication: the relationship with malpractice claims among primary care physicians and surgeons. Journal of the American Medical Association 1997; 277: 553–559.

PART IV

33

The Principle of Fairness

Mr. O'Connell is a 41-year-old man who comes to the office with abdominal cramping, diarrhea and flatulence for the past 24 hours. He returned from Indianapolis last night, after two days at the 500. Yesterday, he ate most of a bag of Corn Chips with Olestra, though not all at once, he said. "I also had some Olestra potato chips. Barbecue. Great tasting. No fat, either."

Dr. Beale examines Mr. O'Connell. His blood pressure is 140/90. He is 67 inches tall and weighs 216 pounds. His abdomen is slightly tender and full, with borborygmi. His stool is hard and heme negative.

FAIRNESS to others, or justice, is the moral basis for managed care. Aiming to improve the health of the population is what makes managed care morally defensible. No one patient is more important or more worthy than any other. All patients deserve equitable and equal care. Population-based health care means care to each according to his or her need and according to the needs of others.

Fairness and population-based care can recall images from *The Lottery,* or from Marx, or from the best run managed care organizations. These pictures are all different and the former is scary, but the true medical and ethical focus of managed care is to improve the health status of a population at risk in a cost-effective manner.

How has fairness changed in this era of managed care? Is fairness more inclusive, kinder and gentler, or is it more exclusive and tougher? Do the haves have more, and the have nots have less, or is the playing field more level than when managed care started?

How has fairness fared?

Fairness *should* **be the most important ethical principle in managed care, especially capitated managed care, but it is not yet.** As mentioned earlier, autonomy and justice have been considered inseparable concepts from ancient times until the present. Why this legacy? Because for one person to say and choose what he or she wants without regard to what others want is unfair if resources come from a common pool.

Yet fairness has been left up to markets in managed care, and fairness does not matter a lot to markets. As policy analyst Emily Friedman has argued, no market is going to worry that rural areas have trouble attracting physicians. Or that distance (i.e., computer-aided) medicine, with the potential to augment physicians, seems even more remote when the server is struck by lightning. No market is going to care if medically indigent inner city residents have a cost-effective primary prevention program, or a Level 1 trauma center or an outpatient mental health program.

Why is fairness a market-mediated commodity? Because the U.S. has neither a strong enough idea of "community"—geographic, spiritual, educational, or occupational—nor a strong enough recognition of interdependence with others to insist that everyone should have a basic level of managed care. Instead of an equitable system that assures an equal level of services to everyone, there is a hodgepodge of temporary alignments.

A managed care organization *should* **care about** *all* **the public's health, not just the health of its members.** But if medicine has to choose between improving the health of the uncovered public and improving the health of the public to which it has access, medicine starts where it can.

The hard and cold facts are that **much of the death and disability in America comes from three behaviors: smoking, eating too many high-fat and low-fiber foods too often, and remaining sedentary.** When added up, one-third of American deaths are directly related to one of these behaviors. The epidemic of tobacco smoking causes 19 percent of all deaths, according to a 1993 JAMA study; 14 percent are caused by dietary patterns and activity levels. Over one-quarter of Americans smoke; an even one-third of Americans are 20 percent or more over ideal body weight.

The most important tool physicians can use to prevent diseases of tobacco and obesity is planning. Lung cancer and heart disease are not diseases of willpower or culpability or age. They are diseases of planning. They take a commitment to quit or change or start, and then a set of tools and skills to execute the change once the commitment is made.

People have to commit on their own, but a minute from a physician about the uncool taste of cigarette kisses to an adolescent with Marlboros in a shirt pocket can help. So can the same minute to a 38-year-old about keeping up with his eight-year-old, or about his own father's angioplasty. The same minute to an apple-shaped 52-year-old reluctant to start estrogen or cut the saturated and trans fats in her diet can make half a lifetime of difference.

Quitting smoking, putting plant foods in the middle of the plate, and integrating regular exercise are not only about personal responsibility. They are also about fairness to other managed care members who must bear the expense—for others' dangerous and disease-breeding choices. Already, some physicians are paying, literally, for their patients who do not attend smoking cessation classes or have their cholesterol levels measured.

The opportunity for medicine is to see the chance for *profession*: the chance to declare aloud a moral compass. Physicians must now show the leadership and vision that have not characterized medicine in the era of managed care. Every time an important issue of fairness has arisen, someone else has taken the lead on it. No physicians are publicly visible leaders on obesity, substance abuse, child abuse, domestic violence, or elder abuse. Clinical research, medical education and postgraduate training are similarly endangered.

These are medical issues that affect the public health which other nonmedical groups have appropriated. With each issue has gone a little bit of power, and with each little bit of power has gone a little more of the sense of what is important to medicine as a profession.

The profession's charge is to acknowledge and reiterate the interrelatedness of individual practices. One physician cannot practice well without the next. Physicians are not isolated, free agents who are justified in gaining for their individual selves whatever they can, without regard for others' interests. Becoming part of a group—even a medical professional group—is hard for some physicians, yet it is more necessary than ever; physicians remain independent of each other at their peril.

In the early 1990s, some states passed laws to protect physicians from avaricious managed care organizations. In the late 1990s, many states are passing laws to protect patients' rights as consumers. Laws that protect patients allow physicians to be better patient advocates. State bills already passed mandate grievance procedures, ban gag clauses, require payment for emergency room visits, limit physician financial incentives, and order open access to some specialists, especially obstetricians and gynecologists.

Though this is a piecemeal approach to justice, it is the American way. Patients took their complaints about choice of physician, bureaucratic inefficiency and coverage to the government. And because politicians want to be re-elected, they listened.

Resource allocation

It is no secret that the real customers of managed care organizations are employers; in most cases, they are the ones who pay for care, and buyer beware. As managed care is regulated, employers will find it less appealing if it is unable to keep costs down. Physicians who have mastered niche areas, such as transplant programs that understand the fair allocation of direly scarce resources, will be ahead of the game.

Solid organ allocation, for example, took a big new step toward fairness after Mickey Mantle's liver transplant. If donor livers, kidneys and hearts go to the sickest person first, they have the least chance of succeeding. A less sick person who might survive the transplant will not have had a chance. So, the new triage reasoning goes, why not give the liver to the person who is most likely to survive?

The United Network for Organ Sharing (UNOS) now agrees: With some exceptions, the liver should go to the person most likely to survive. But UNOS' recent change in its allocation rules, still under negotiation, appropriately disrupts what philosopher E. Haavi Morreim calls the "rule of rescue" mentality that bloated health care into a wasteful system of unnecessary operations and medications and begat managed care.

The rule of rescue is precisely the opposite of managed care's ambition to be fair to all its members. Rescue makes the least sense when the resource cannot be divided and remain effective and when there are others to consider.

Utilization is also the real issue for prescription drug plans. Prescription programs are popular among patients for a reason: They are a strong financial incentive to patients to join managed care. Is the primary goal still cost-containment? If physicians achieve a 90 percent generic substitution rate will some prescriptions for generic digoxin slip through the physician's pad to the pharmacist? And should therapeutic substitution be prohibited?

Therapeutic substitutions allow pharmacists to substitute, for example, a less expensive ACE-inhibitor for the actually prescribed one. At best this can cause confusion for a patient, as dosages and effects may have been explained in the office; at worst, a patient can take the substituted medication and have no relief of symptoms and an adverse reaction.

Usually, therapeutic substitution poses only inconvenience—something patients happily attempt to reduce in signing up for managed care, and usually do not encounter a lot of again unless they are unlucky enough to need a referral out-of-plan or an off-formulary medication.

But sometimes utilization decisions about prescription drugs and other treatment must be appealed—when a patient's personal medical interests are threatened or when medical danger is imminent. Patients may not always perceive this danger in the same way as do their physicians, and have strong financial incentives to accept whatever drug is substituted. Being better informed about managed care terms can only help patients get what they (and their employer) paid for.

Justice in managed care: the road ahead

"It's the corn chips and the potato chips," Dr. Beale tells Mr. O'Connell. "Make sure you drink eight to 10 cups of water today and tomorrow. You need to eat two whole yellow or red vegetables every day, and a green leafy vegetable every day for at least a month—not just a spinach leaf either—a whole head of quick-steamed broccoli, with lemon and garlic. Also a multivitamin with D, E, A and K in it. Take this slip and let's measure your cholesterol. Come back next week and we'll discuss your tests and some ways to reduce your weight."

There is hope for justice in managed care if disease prevention, duty to others and social mission achieve a more prominent place at the managed care planning table.

What can clinicians do to promote fairness to patients and others, including themselves, in managed care?

1. **Acknowledge that the conflict between fidelity to an individual patient and the greatest good for the greatest number is part of managed care.** Ask patients to do the same. This action emphasizes organizational and social accountability.

2. **Become an expert on at least one preventive topic:** obesity management, smoking cessation, physical fitness, alcoholism treatment, public safety, vaccination, stress management, domestic violence prevention. Remember that every effort made to prevent illness improves clinicians' ability to provide for others and extends the available capitated resources.

3. **Be prepared to work largely for incentives, not just for salary.** Some sacrifice will be required to keep physicians together as a profession and as collegial groups. Volume incentives without modification for disease severity are counterproductive. Incentives that are proportionate to effort, nonpunitive, and that improve care quality are worthwhile.

4. **Make sure that the patient actually wants an appeal if treatment is unfairly denied.** Review the reasons for treatment, payment alternatives and other choices. Be realistic about the benefits of treatment and the risks of nontreatment. Consider a time-limited trial of treatment, if feasible.

5. **The person who is most assertive in seeking care usually gets what he or she wants. This may not be fair, but it's true. Advise patients to insist and persist if faced with a denial of treatment:** *A physician's recommendation, even if denied as medically unnecessary, is strong medicine.* Tell the patient that he or she has the right to seek treatment on his or her own in the event of a disagreement, and if possible, get others to pay for it later. Patients can use their employee benefits administrator, demand re-evaluation from the managed care review board, write the medical director, and document clinical reasons for the denial and the names, titles, dates and times in conversations, and calls never returned. Complaints to a disease advocacy group, local legislators, and the state insurance department may all yield a settlement.

6. **Learn about legally established grievance and appeals rights, or advocates provided by a consumer protection agency or the state attorney general. Avoiding**

litigation and arbitration is also a goal here, as these processes put most patients at a disadvantage relative to the managed care organization. The poor, the powerless, the uneducated, the uninsured, the underinsured, and the home bound elderly do not have access to an attorney or to the media, and will end up being squashed unless they know about and use their formal grievance and appeals rights.

3 4

Smoking, Slimming and Seat Belts: Is Public Health and Preventive Medicine a Responsibility of Managed Care?

MONEY doesn't buy health, never mind love. The United States spends more than any other country on health care, but our average lifespan is lower than most in Western Europe and Canada. Our major causes of death and disability are related to how much we smoke, how much and what we eat and how much we exercise. Coronary disease, emphysema, diabetes, osteoarthritis and many cancers are largely "life-style diseases."

What changes has medicine made in the past that could support future changes in smoking, obesity and seat belt/helmet use? Can incentives to physicians make public health part of an increasingly private managed care mission?

Changing behavior

To start, physicians have, in one case, already changed behavior. In the 1960s it was still acceptable for doctors to smoke cigarettes; in the 1990s, after millions of cases of chronic bronchitis and cardiovascular disease, nearly all U.S. physicians have quit.

Physicians have changed ideas about how to counsel patients. In the early 1960s, for example, 90 percent of physicians in one survey thought it was unethical to tell cancer patients their diagnoses. By the late 1970s, only 10 percent of physicians thought so.

There are three areas in which I believe physicians must now institute further change in what they tell patients: smoking, obesity and seat belts.

Smoking

Rikers Island did something in 1996 that no managed care organization has yet been able to do. The correctional institution induced its population, guards included, to quit smoking. It's apparently illegal to smoke in public places in New York, and that includes jails. How ironic that one of the only groups in America guaranteed access to health care—inmates—is also guaranteed no danger from secondhand smoke.

How toxic cigarettes are, how early teen-agers start and how much tobacco drives up health costs are not at issue. Joe Camel billboards, Marlboro gift catalogues and full-page *New York Times* ads addressed to Nabisco stockholders work against patients.

Yet patients can quit if they have a plan. Nicotine gum recently went to over-the-counter status, and so will nicotine patches. Together with brief, nonjudgmental encouragement from a doctor and regular support groups, these medical bridges do work. Patients who quit smoking and have several negative random plasma cotinine levels should have expanded wellness benefits, reduced premiums or both.

Obesity

In the 1960s, Helen Worth's *Cooking Without Recipes* declared that "canned vegetables offer more food value than market vegetables." In the 1990s, "organic and locally grown" clean food from farmers' markets and health food stores suggests quality, safety, health and flavor.

Most Americans' health problems come from too much food, not too little. Today, 34 percent of adults are 20 percent or more over ideal body weight. And too many medical schools still teach nutrition simply as vitamin and mineral deficiencies.

At least one group, Cambridge's Oldways Preservation and Exchange Trust, wants to help. With the World Health Organization, Oldways researches the traditional diets of cultures that spend much less on health care and have much less obesity, heart disease and cancer than we do. Its Mediterranean and Asian "diet pyramids" are lauded by the USDA; its Latin American and vegetarian diet pyramids have just been released.

A worldwide scientific consensus on what constitutes healthy eating patterns was echoed by the revised 1995 U.S. Dietary Guidelines. But consensus doesn't control eating habits. Twenty years of testing an insoluble fat substitute called Olestra have resulted in new Pringles potato chips, despite enough diarrhea in clinical trials to require package warnings. And because our eating habits haven't improved, millions took phen/fen, two appetite suppressants with side effects that cancel each other out. The dyad is now history, after a brief run at the "most prescribed futile combination" award.

The Oldways models are important, and the new dietary guidelines are steps in the right direction. Dangerous diet drugs that can cause valvular damage and Olestra's "anal seepage" are steps in the wrong direction.

What hasn't been tried to treat obesity? Incentives to physicians and nurses to counsel, and to patients to take

that counsel. Physicians who help obese patients lose 10 percent of body fat and keep it off for two years should be rewarded financially. Patients who do the same for two years or more should see reduced premiums. Food, cooking and exercise belong in the discussion between clinicians and patients as much as do potassium levels for patients on diuretics.

Seat belts

In 1996, the U.S. Department of Transportation released a report analyzing more than 800,000 traffic collisions that took place in seven states in 1990. Only two-thirds of the drivers involved used seat belts, but $68 million would have been saved if all had used them. Hospital costs for unbelted drivers were $5,000 higher (55 percent higher) than for unbelted drivers.

Most people are shielded from the real cost of accidents as they are from the real cost of health care. On average, people pay only about 15 percent out of pocket, according to the *American Medical News*; the rest is picked up by auto insurers and others. Like other patients, accident victims seldom see the real cost of hospitalization, paid by insurers or managed care organizations and ultimately by employers or others in the form of premiums.

Slimming down, stopping smoking and wearing seat belts would probably have more impact on health care costs and quality of life than any other three behavior changes. Managed care should have the courage and vision to promote them as treatment for the illnesses they engender. Physicians should lead this health effort because patients listen when physicians counsel about life-style. **Smoking, food and seat belt choices are power—economic power. We can help patients unleash this power by encouraging personal responsibility, the very foundation of morality.**

Just as Oldways wants people to "vote with their forks," doctors should vote with their incentives. In addition to those mentioned, these should reflect the number of referrals to stop-smoking classes and the documentation of seat belt and helmet advice (even in an unrelated office visit) and of spoken tips about diet, fat and exercise. Patients already have incentives to stay within network and take formulary medications: They should also have incentives to prevent disease.

Making public health a private business might just make enough room to include people who have been left out of managed care—the uninsured—for every patient's good.

For Further Reading:

1. Breslow L. Public health and managed care: a California perspective. Health Affairs 1996; 15(1):92–99.
2. La Puma J. Help your patients eat their way to health. Managed Care—A Guide for Physicians 1996 June; 47–52.
3. Law M, Tang JL. An analysis of the effectiveness of interventions intended to help people stop smoking. Archives of Internal Medicine 1995; 155: 1933–1941.
4. McGinnis JM, Foegge WH. Actual causes of death in the United States. Journal of the American Medical Association 1993; 270:2207–2212.

3 5

Ethics Catches Up to Law: What Is Most Fair for All?

THICAL ISSUES in managed care arise with the overlap of ethics and economics. Ethics and law also overlap,
and courts have been changing the way they think about
ethical issues.

Managed care plans, especially HMOs, thus far have had a re-
markable degree of immunity from liability, but physicians who
are part of plans may still be exposed. The reason? Medical ethics
is just starting to catch up with medical law in considering clinical
economic issues.

Judge-made insurance

So far, courts generally have ruled in favor of patients
against managed care plans if treatment limitations were
somehow unclear or decidedly unfair. In *Warne v. Lincoln National* (Fourth Judicial District Court of Idaho, No. 96932, 1994),
the HMO had advertised coverage for organ transplants in its pro-
motional brochures, but dropped coverage in the actual contract.
Mr. Warne needed a liver transplant, but Lincoln refused to pay.
The Warnes raised the funds themselves, and the patient had the
operation, but died. Mrs. Warne later sued Lincoln National for its
refusal. The jury award was $26.8 million.

Cases like these emphasize what philosopher Haavi Morreim cites as **"judge-made insurance"—occasional, nearly random episodes of compassion from a court or jury that recognize the relative vulnerability of an individual HMO member, against which the resources of an insurance entity loom large.**

Cases like these also call into question the patient's fiscal responsibilities to other members. What are those responsibilities? Actually, members pay for each other's care in a managed care organization. Yet patients operate on the principle of "me first."

Patient self-determination has been the dominant ethical principle in American medicine for almost half a century. Myriad conventional and alternative choices in health care remind us that patient autonomy is not going away. Perhaps, however, it should be brought into balance with other important ethical principles.

Justice, or fairness, is one such principle. Autonomy and justice historically have been considered together, from Plato and Aristotle forward, because for one person to say and choose what he or she wants without regard to what others want is unfair—especially if resources come from a common pool.

Autonomy and justice may be coming together again. Several legal cases suggest that we need the wisdom of more than one ethical principle to have an ethical managed care future. For example, in *Fuja v. Benefit Trust Life Insurance Co.* (18 F.3d 1407 7th Cir, 1994), a woman with metastatic breast cancer was referred for bone marrow transplantation. The transplant was denied, as the patient's insurance contract specifically prohibited experimental procedures. The Seventh Circuit Court supported Benefit Trust, seeing the issue as one of contract interpretation.

Contractual fairness is just one type of fairness. There is also distributive justice *(to each according to his need)*; **egalitarian justice** *(to each according to what similar others receive)*; **and utilitarian justice** *(to each according to what's best for all).*

Judging clinical cases by the wording of a contract can integrate fairness and autonomy, but it's neither the only way to do so nor a generous one. Sadly, employers who offer employees health care of any kind must be as concerned with making their budgets as with helping their employees care for themselves and their families.

A different approach to integrating fairness with autonomy is to try to be as scientific as possible about medicine. In *Barnett v. Kaiser Foundation Health Plan, Inc.* (32 F.3d 413, 9th Cir 1994), a man with e-antigen positive hepatitis was referred for transplantation. The procedure was denied by the Kaiser Foundation Health Plan liver transplant advisory board because, the board reportedly said, the highly infectious disease would cause the transplant to fail and was therefore contraindicated. Mr. Barnett paid privately for the procedure and then sued. The Ninth U.S. Circuit Court of Appeals found in Kaiser's favor. Medical criteria, it decided, were a valid way to make medical judgments about efficacy and benefit. Physicians are the appropriate people to make allocation decisions about such resources.

Trade-offs between the individual and the group have to be made, the court said, and providing benefits to as many plan members as possible was Kaiser's job, though it would be inappropriate to make medical decisions based solely on saving Kaiser money.

Just as in fee-for-service or salaried medicine, the safest ethical and legal position for the physician is still to be an individual patient advocate first. Although this individual advocacy may run contrary to the details of the contract a patient or his employer signed and to principles of justice and population-based health, personal advocacy is still what individual patients expect. Whether they *should* expect that individual advocacy from a physician is a different, harder question.

Physicians, ethicists and attorneys are beginning to address cases that shift the discussion from what a physician owes individual patients to his or her responsibilities to all managed care organization patients. With this shift comes the fundamental question: Doesn't our society owe some level of medical care to all its citizens? Managed care organizations, for their own communities and at their most noble, can answer.

For Further Reading:

1. Clancy CM, Brody H. Managed care: Jekyll or Hyde? Journal of the American Medical Association 1995; 273:338–339.
2. Miles SH, Parker P. Men, women and health insurance. New England Journal of Medicine 1997; 336:218–221.
3. Ware JE Jr, Bayliss MS, Rogers WH, Kosinski M, Tarlov AR. Differences in 4 year health outcomes for elderly and poor, chronically ill patients treated in HMO and fee-for-service systems: results from the Medical Outcomes Study. Journal of the American Medical Association 1996; 276:1039–1047.

36

Mickey Mantle's
Liver Transplant:
Is Organ Allocation Fair?

MORE CANCER was found in the body of baseball great Mickey Mantle a few weeks after his well-publicized liver transplant. Had the lung cancer been detected earlier, we are told, the ailing superstar would not have been a transplant candidate. But even as we wished Mantle well, we recognized that his operation, given the doctors' knowledge at the time it was performed, already raised key questions of triage and fairness for the medical community.

Several managed care organizations have refused to pay for transplants, calling the procedure "experimental." A number of these cases have gone to court, and generally they have been decided in the patient's favor. But by that time, it has usually been too late.

Mickey Mantle reportedly had alcoholic cirrhosis, hepatitis C and liver cancer. He also reportedly was critically ill and 63 years old. These are news reports data; who knows the real facts? While there are probably experimental protocols that include patients who have liver cancer, it's unlikely that any experimental transplant protocol includes medically ravaged people with three fatal liver diseases. Yet Mantle got into a transplant center, and once there, was ranked on the list of waiting patients kept by the United Network for Organ Sharing (UNOS).

What is the real ethical issue here? Is it a dire scarcity of livers, and the way they are distributed through UNOS? Or is it the "experimental" nature of therapeutic innovation in surgery and access to that innovation in the first place?

Dire scarcity means that a resource is either absolutely absent or so rare that it cannot be divided and remain effective—one kidney, an intensive care unit bed, a single dose of penicillin. **Few resources are direly scarce in the United States, but a donor liver is one of them.** There are approximately 4,600 people on the UNOS national waiting list, and they are ranked by blood type and degree of urgency: status 1, 2, 3, 4.

Direly scarce resources are often triaged. The military system of war-time triage dictates that the sickest person does not get the resource, and neither does the least sick person. Instead, the patient in the middle gets it, because the overall goal of treatment is to return patients to health as soon as possible so they can resume fighting.

Who gets scarce organs?

In U.S. civilian life, the first livers available for transplant, however direly scarce, are not given to the patients most likely to survive. They are given to patients who are dying or acutely ill—those in the hospital, often in the ICU. These are patients who can no longer wait for the only available treatment, and who also have the best chance of dying with a now spent, still precious resource.

Why give a direly scarce organ first to someone who is *least* likely to survive? Would it be right for UNOS to make a policy of distributing its direly scarce livers to patients who are *most* likely to survive? Should managed care organizations distribute livers differently than UNOS does?

The UNOS system reflects American medicine's "rule of rescue" mentality and the public's expectation that nearly every medical circumstance can be controlled. When someone is ill, the physician's job is to pull him out of it. When someone is dying, our job is to reverse the process. When someone has done injury to himself, our job is to repair it.

The "fix-it" philosophy

This "fix-it" philosophy is necessarily retrospective and focuses on treatment, rather than on prevention. It is the precise opposite of the managed care philosophy, which emphasizes health promotion and personal responsibility and de-emphasizes trials of expensive, experimental interventions.

What is experimental treatment? The answer to this question varies from one managed care organization to another and has been the subject of several suits. No matter how it's defined, "experimental treatment" is a misnomer. When a procedure is performed, it is intended either as research, to gather generalizable knowledge for the good of future patients, or as therapy, to cure, palliate or restore for the good of a particular patient.

Philosopher Stan Reiser has used the term "crossover therapy" to bridge the gap between research and standard treatment. [Health Affairs 1994; 13(3):127–136.] Research protocols, writes Reiser, are plagued by uncertainty and inflexibility, even more than standard treatment. Standard treatment relies upon established medical indications, specified outcomes of care, standardized requirements for practice, and articulated criteria for training and certification. Crossover therapy (such as liver transplantation for a patient with cirrhosis, hepatitis, and cancer, perhaps) has elements of both research and treatment.

Especially in surgery, crossover therapy often seems inseparable from just plain treatment, from the patient's perspective. Although there are excellent examples of prospective trials of surgical innovation—segmental liver transplantation in children, for example—these are too rare, and not the norm. What the patient gets, even if there is no standard therapy available, is individualized by the physician at the patient's side.

Certainly an individual approach based on the patient's

need is the best approach for therapy that is not direly scarce, and when limited resources are not an issue. But livers are scarce, and in managed care organizations resources are especially limited.

The celebrity factor

Access to heart and liver transplant protocols, like other types of access to specialized treatment, is greased by the ability to pay. Can celebrity and positive publicity serve as proxies for the ability to pay and reasons to bend the scientific or ethical rules? For someone of Mantle's stature, they certainly can. Protocols, of course, do not make exceptions for celebrities—but people do. And getting into the transplant center and on the protocol was exceptional.

Sympathy is apropos for a 63-year-old man with three fatal liver diseases and a very short life expectancy, and Mickey Mantle should have had the best treatment medicine can offer. So should every other 63-year-old.

Mantle's case presents an opportunity for physicians to stand on the ground of fairness when our ill patients are denied access to expensive treatment that is "experimental." We can now use Mantle's demonstration of privilege to gain some for other patients.

For Further Reading:

1. Hauptman PJ, O'Connor KJ. Procurement and allocation of solid organs for transplantation. New England Journal of Medicine 1997; 336:422–431.
2. Moss AH, Siegler M. Should alcoholics compete equally for liver transplantation? Journal of the American Medical Association 1991; 265(10):1295–1298.
3. Steinbrook R. Allocating livers—devising a fair system. New England Journal of Medicine 1997; 336:436–438.

3 7

Satisfying Managed Care Patients Through Ethics Consultation

S ATISFACTION RESEARCH is hot. Patient satisfaction surveys are easy to do, and tie happily and immediately into the health care operating strategy of the '90s (continuous quality improvement through total quality management). They also can be added to whatever framework an organization has for collecting data. But the shift toward managed care is part of a new consumerism in medicine, and it brings up different ethical problems. Patients seem to accept population-based health care, for example, only as it affords them access to the care they as individuals want.

While patients are satisfied with the costs and paper work of managed care, they are relatively less satisfied with access to treatment. Once denied care, few patients can make their own case in person. Fewer physicians feel effective in trying to help.

Satisfaction with hands-on, inpatient ethics consultation by trained committee members and consultants is high among physicians who request it. As a field, ethics consultation has grown, but it is unsure of how to respond to the shift towards managed care and with economic issues in medicine.

Should ethics consultation continue to be provided as a clinical service, primarily for physicians who need help

with a "do not resuscitate" order, or ventilator with-drawal? Should consultation try to save money as part of quality improvement, pleasing payers and employers? Or should ethics consultation reinvent itself in this time of tight resources and concern about values, and become a patient advocacy and quality mechanism?

Satisfaction: a quick review

Satisfied patients have better compliance rates, participate in their own treatment more and say they are more likely to come back. Patients who are older and who are female tend to be more satisfied with hospital care and physicians than patients who are younger or male.

The Boston-based Picker Institute's "patient-centered questions" about satisfaction focus on seven areas that matter most to patients. They are:

- Respect for patient values, preferences and expressed needs;
- Coordination, integration and information flow;
- Communication, information and education;
- Physical comfort;
- Emotional support and alleviation of fear and anxiety;
- Involvement of family and friends; and
- Overall satisfaction and recommendation to others.

The Picker research shows that patients value commu-nication of information about health or medical treatment more than physicians do, while physicians believe their pa-tients value privacy, courtesy and overall helpfulness.

Satisfaction with both physicians and inpatient care is still gen-erally high. The same is true for many managed care and indem-nity plans, making discrimination between patient-pleasing characteristics difficult.

Satisfaction with inpatient care seems to depend on two sets of factors: hotel-like services and medical/physician care. Attendant and staff courtesy, promptness, waiting time, food and food service all affect patients' stated willingness to return to an institution. **Satisfaction with physician care depends on perceived technical competence and interpersonal skills. Specialists rate higher than generalists in technical competence. The longer a physician spends with a patient, the more highly his/her interpersonal skills are rated.**

Many believe that the health system has changed so fundamentally that a new focus for ethics is needed, and that focus has to do with different components of provider and patient satisfaction than have been previously studied. For example, physicians who actually are protected against liability exposure, and who do receive prompt assistance from a colleague trained and available to help with ethical dilemmas will be highly satisfied. Patients who have increased access to and education about treatment and treatment options will be the same.

There is another way for ethics consultation to go. It could change its goals to pure patient advocacy, and do so through standard-setting. Marion Danis, M.D., has advocated the need for "ethical standards, just as there are standards to assure quality in the delivery of the technical aspects of medical care. . . . The patient should also be able to expect that access to care, informed consent and the right to refuse treatment are ethical standards that will be met" (Journal of Clinical Ethics 1994; 5(2):159–162).

The Joint Committee on Accreditation of Healthcare Organizations has new standards for institutions in patient rights (to access, treatment and respect) and in organizational ethics. The National Committee for Quality Assurance is considering standards too. The JCAHO's standards require hospital and network codes of ethics to address financial conflicts of interest with clinical decision-making. The AMA is moving toward standard-setting in ethics for the profession as a whole, and the American Hospital Association is emphasizing member corporate ethics in 1998.

Ethics consultation should now address the distinct outpatient and inpatient issues of coverage, rationing and triage that managed care raises. Ethics consultation may need to assume a role that is even more strongly and publicly oriented.

It should address managed care resource allocation decisions, and help to create guidelines concerning ethical issues.

New goals for consultation

Ethics consultation should now attempt to discover systematically the ethical problems that patients have within hospitals and managed care, and to reshape, align and then test ways in which ethics services can satisfy patients. Patients need a new, access-oriented advocacy, and ethics consultants should be available—and paid to be available—to colleagues and patients to appeal decisions, work with quality and utilization management, and help hospital and physician organizations create ethical guidance for cases and clinical policies. Ethics consultation should seek to become a mechanism by which managed care restores its tarnished credibility with patients.

Future research should focus on ways to improve demonstrated patient dissatisfaction; to anticipate ethical dilemmas using proactive, standardized quality management approaches; to register an ability to meet practical ethical guidelines; to diminish futile care; to improve access to beneficial care; and to study different ways of achieving each of these clinical goals.

For Further Reading:

1. Agich GJ. Authority in ethics consultation. Journal of Law, Medicine and Ethics 1995; 23(3):273–283.
2. Fox E, Arnold RM. Evaluating outcomes in ethics consultation research. Journal of Clinical Ethics 1996; 7(2):127–138.
3. La Puma J, Darling CA, Stocking CB, Siegler M. Community hospital ethics consultation: evaluation and comparison with a university hospital service. American Journal of Medicine 1992; 92:346–351.

3 8

What to Expect From Your Hospital's Ethics Program

IN SOME DIFFICULT CASES, the hospital ethicist can be as important as the primary care physician. Yet even with today's proliferation of ethics committees, consultation services and programs, help is not available to many physicians who must negotiate with a disagreeing family, interpret an unclear advance directive, or write a portable "do not resuscitate" order.

What should physicians expect from their hospitals' ethics programs, as managed care systems change institutions from revenue generators to cost centers? How can ethics programs offer services that patients and physicians in a particular institution actually need *and* that the Joint Commission on Accreditation of Healthcare Organizations (JCAHO) has required since 1995? And what are some of the newer ethical issues physicians encounter in managed care?

Institutional motivation

Hospitals have significant new motivations to strengthen and improve their ethics committees and programs. **JCAHO's 1998 accreditation standards emphasize patient rights to access, treatment and respect, and organizational ethics. They re-**

quire institutions to implement "an ethics process to deal with ethical issues." Among those issues, the JCAHO lists:

Forgoing life-sustaining treatment;
Resolving disagreements in care decisions;
Forgoing resuscitation;
Decision-making by surrogates;
Deciding to participate in research;
Respecting patient confidentiality, privacy, security complaints and communication; and
Formulating advance directives.

The JCAHO also has new ethics, rights and responsibilities standards for health care networks. Since 1994, its network ethics standards have required "an effective mechanism for member involvement" and covered almost the same list of issues, plus three unique ones in 1998.

Independent appeal mechanisms, outside of plan control, are on the way. Some managed care organizations seek accreditation from the National Committee on Quality Assurance (NCQA), and as dilemmas of billing, coding, referring and honesty have been publicized, the NCQA has looked harder at numbers of grievances, appeals and complaints. Though accreditation is voluntary, major employers want plans that have it. Only 20 percent of organizations that undergo review by NCQA are fully accredited, and approximately 15 percent are denied accreditation.

Physicians should expect good service from their institutional ethics program. They should look for five basic functions in such a program: education, clinical service, research, community involvement and policymaking. The most well-established ethics committees often have all five. Successful programs nearly always have a well-respected clinician leader. Goals, objectives, timeline, mission and vision are clearly spelled out. Issues in organizational ethics, such as managing staff requests, interpreting the required code, and disclosing ownership of referred services, are on progressive committee radar screens.

Getting down to cases

Case-based education is an effective way to learn clinical ethics and to become involved in an ethics committee program. Cases are familiar territory, and because the knowledge base involved is highly pragmatic and material abundant, case-based education is a good place to start.

Clinical service requires a clinician or clinical consulting team with skill, availability and training. Seeing the patient is critical— and often omitted. Yet case consultation can be an area of excellence, with minimum training and maximum benefit, if institutional sponsorship and support are adequate.

Research functions may be simple record-keeping, for financial, professional and social purposes, or may involve quality improvement, risk management and utilization committees.

Community involvement in discussions of institutional ethical issues, from advance directives to genetic screening to choice of physician to respect for and care of the dying, will ensure the relevance of an ethics program to the community overall.

Policymaking, especially in areas in which ethics and economics overlap, will be the forte of the excellent ethics committee of the 21st century. Managed care embodies the overlap of ethics and economics, and physicians who assist patients, families and colleagues with ethical problems can bring bedside issues to the boardroom in an immediate, realistic way.

Reasons to consult

What are the most common reasons physicians currently ask for inpatient ethics service? Data from ethics consultation services in community hospitals show that physicians most often ask questions about:

Withdrawing or withholding treatment;
Resolving a disagreement between health care professionals, patients and families;
Deciding about resuscitation status;

Evaluating a patient's decision-making capacity;
Assessing legal issues;
Meeting professional responsibility; and
Formulating, interpreting and implementing advance
directives.

These issues almost parallel the JCAHO's list and show its inpatient orientation. Institutions that design and implement educational, clinical, research and policy programs around the issues that concern their own hospital staff and patients will be headed in the right direction.

How do the ethical issues differ in managed care?

In the *inpatient setting*, newer issues encountered by clinicians arise from the changes in the doctor-patient relationship. They include:

Conflicts of billing, coding and referring;
Questions about "marginal" care and who should pay
for it; and
Appealing financial constraints on a patient's treatment.

In the *outpatient setting*, ethical issues are common, yet essentially unexplored and nearly undocumented. **Outpatient ethics concerns three general areas: conflicting loyalties, communication, and professional and social responsibilities.** These areas are now partially covered by the JCAHO standards unique to networks. Timely grievance resolution is required, but so is "complying with a recommended treatment" and "cooperating with health care providers." Accountability, here we come!

What to do? **Physicians should discuss their own ethics cases in established, accepted forums for education and management.** Dilemmas of coverage, choice, adherence and access, when described by an illustrative case, will challenge the most creative of us to identify, analyze and resolve them. They'll also help to catch the accreditor's eye.

Institutions need physician leadership to identify and analyze ethical problems, especially as managed care becomes the primary way hospitals finance and deliver care. Physicians should participate in and help to lead ethics committees and consultation services, whether sponsored by a hospital, a managed care organization, a health care network, a medical staff, or all four. A strong, well-run ethics program can meet medical and institutional expectations by delivering first-class service when it is least expected: in difficult clinical cases.

For Further Reading:

1. Corsino BV. Bioethics committees and JCAHO Patients' Rights standards: a question of balance. Journal of Clinical Ethics 1996; 7(2):177–181.
2. Fletcher JC. Responding to JCAHO standards: everybody's business. Journal of Clinical Ethics 1996; 7(2):182–183.
3. Pastin M. The medical ethics committee: dinosaur or phoenix? Health Systems Review 1996; 29(6):15–16,19.

Managed Care Ethics: CME

Prepared by Hatherleigh Press

How to earn CME using this section: The dual mission of a Hatherleigh CME Book is to provide medical professionals with a review of authoritative, practical information that illuminates the common and challenging clinical issues they encounter in their daily work, and to include with that information an exam that enables them to earn Category I credit toward the recertification of their license.

This book can be used to earn continuing medical education credits via the CME Appendix. The boldfaced sentences throughout the book highlight the learning points. To earn CME credits using this book, simply call Hatherleigh to order a quiz response form using the toll-free number, 1-800-367-2550. Hatherleigh representatives will inform you of the options available to you as a participant in one of our CME programs.

Learning objectives: In this book, the author examines ethical questions raised by late 20th century changes in health care delivery—in particular, managed care. Ethical principles that govern care have not changed, however. These include autonomy, accountability, integrity, beneficence and fairness.

Autonomy, the active involvement of the patient in his or her medical choices, has been on the rise, but before long it may be balanced with the principle of fairness. That each patient should have the best medical care available is countered with the consideration of what is adequate and available for all people, as resources are inevitably limited. The obligation to care for those who cannot afford care of any kind and the place of marginal and futile care are considered.

Accountability for one's own health and for adherence to negotiated medical plans is highlighted. In particular, a new emphasis must be placed on educating patients to seek and use accurate information, including ways to prevent disease that can be controlled with behavioral and lifestyle changes.

The individual physician's professional allegiance to a patient is now complemented by the need for managed care organizations to model integrity and compassion towards patients as well. These virtues have important risk management and legal implications.

Beneficence, doing what is good for the patient, often requires physicians and patients to work together to see that proper diagnostic and treatment measures are given, even when faced with treatment delays or denials. Fairness, or treating each patient within the limits of available resources, is a moral standard for managed care, against which employers will judge it. Paradoxically, many employees are offered no health plan at all.

The author offers guidelines for approaching the issue of confidentiality, which is assuming a number of new risks, not the least of which is the ready availability of computerized records to many different people. Suggestions are also offered about ways in which physicians can maintain meaningful personal relationships with patients in a world in which the doctor-patient interaction has become increasingly impersonal and patients can and do change doctors to reduce costs.

In 1998, the Joint Committee on the Accreditation of Healthcare Organizations (JCAHO) emphasized clinical ethics and required institutions to have a "functioning process to address ethical issues." Among these are forgoing life-sustaining treatment; resolving disagreement in care decision; forgoing resuscitation decision-making by surrogates; deciding to participate in research; procuring/donating organs; respecting patient confidentiality, privacy and communication; and formulating advance directives. It is within the framework of these requirements and their outpatient equivalents—treatment, coverage, patient access, financial incentives and disclosure, gatekeeping and referrals to specialists—that the author addresses ethical issues and outlines the value of consultation when physicians are faced with particularly difficult dilemmas that touch upon ethical issues.

1. **The principle of autonomy supports:**
   A. The idea that patients should make all decisions relevant to their treatment on their own
   B. The physician's right to assist a patient to commit suicide
   C. Shared decision-making involving the physician, the patient and, when appropriate, the patient's family
   D. The concept that all patients should be treated equally

2. **According to the author, the real issue about confidentiality *within the managed care context* is:**
   A. A growing tendency for information to be leaked to the press by treating professionals when the patient is a celebrity

B. Patient information contained on an employer's database that could be used to influence a patient's career, his or her ability to get life insurance, and other important life considerations

C. Considerably less concern on the part of physicians to keep patients' information confidential

D. None of the above

3. Physicians can honor a patient's autonomy by all except which of the following tactics:

A. Honor autonomy when it is about personal choices, such as being sure the patient has not been misinformed by information presented via public media

B. Solicit patient preference by asking for his/her opinion and understanding, noting the words the patient uses to express these

C. Always conferring with the patient's family to be sure they agree with the patient's choices

D. Utilize a separate, advance planning office visit to discuss *palliative care*

4. Which of the following statements is correct?

A. In managed care, the principle of autonomy is diametrically opposed to the principle of accountability

B. Patients should not be held accountable for managing and preventing disease of any sort, even those which could be largely within their own control

C. In the managed care setting, doctors should continue to be the patient's advocate, even when appeals through traditional medical and administrative structures have failed and a patient's medical interests remain threatened

D. In managed care, patients are more likely to be overtreated than undertreated because of concern by the various plans' managers that they may face malpractice liability

5. The reasons offered by the author for the emphasis on practice guidelines in managed care programs include all *except* which of the following?

A. Financial incentives to limit treatment

B. The growing emphasis on patient accountability

C. Population versus individual medical care

D. Shifts in the location and character of practice

6. Which of the following items is *not* one of the components of quality cited by the RAND Corporation's Medical Outcomes Study?

A. Financial and organizational accessibility

B. Continuity and comprehensiveness

C. Strict employment of established diagnostic and treatment guidelines

D. Interpersonal and technical accountability

7. Which of the following is *not* cited by the author as a way for doctors to become more personal physicians, modeling the virtues necessary for patients to succeed in managed care?

A. Arrange for an ethics consultation for every patient one sees

B. Negotiate more, both with patients and those who monitor treatment

C. Schedule more time for medical and financial discussions with patients

D. Learn more about colleagues' approaches to problems

8. To make managed care work ethically, any plan's management should:

A. Demonstrate respect for physicians' professional dedication to the care of the sick

B. Refute cost containment as the most important goal, the mantra, of managed care

C. Invite broad participation in policy-making

D. Ignore dual role conflicts (the interests of the patient vs. the profitability of the organization), favoring the company's goals first most of the time

9. Integrity, another ethical principle, is:

A. Always personal, never organizational

B. Nice to see in organizations, but hardly a business necessity

C. Organizational as well as individual, and, in managed care, its presence or absence is seen in how management relates to itself, to the physicians it employs, and to the patients it serves

D. All of the above

10. Which of the following skills is *not* one cited for physicians to acquire in order to succeed in managed care?

A. How to read contracts and negotiate carefully

B. Maintain a very strong professional individuality vs. working well in teams

C. How to continue to draw one's self-esteem from the relational stimulation and society of medicine

D. Arrive at a way to evaluate just how much profit the principle of fairness really allows anyone in the system

11. In order to bolster organizational integrity and maintain their own, physicians can:

A. Avoid assuming any management responsibilities

B. Create an ethics mechanism to address hard choices

C. Refrain from talking about money with patients

D. Make clear to all their patients that they must always follow the strict guidelines of the managed care company with whom they are affiliated, whether those are in any patient's best health interests or not

12. **Which of the following statements is correct?**
    A. Whenever a physician wants a little more time with a patient than is allowed, he/she should never hesitate to make up an additional diagnosis to cover the extra time, e.g. adding a fictitious neuropathy to an otherwise uncomplicated diagnosis of diabetes IIB
    B. Hispanic-Americans and Korean-Americans consistently prefer not to have families involved in medical decision-making
    C. In one study, 86 percent of Navaho health providers and patients disapproved of the federally mandated Patient Self-Determination Act which requires doctors to tell an ill patient that he/she may refuse treatment because doing so might bring on loss of hope
    D. All of the above

13. **To practice more effectively in culturally diverse managed care, one should:**
    A. Emphasize personal respect, e.g. using proper family names
    B. Use nonfamily interpreters
    C. Ask patients if they want to know their diagnoses and make decisions, or if they'd like someone else involved to do it
    D. All of the above

14. **Which of the following statements is correct?**
    A. There are few ethical considerations associated with the cost of care near the end of life
    B. Ethical issues raised by underwriting (an insurance term defined as the process of selecting risk) include the language used to speak about patients, such as "customers" or "loss ratios"
    C. Capitation for the care of Medicare patients places many physicians at a much lower financial risk than capitation for younger populations
    D. None of the above

15. **According to the author, three ways to attempt to minimize the possibility of distortion resulting from financial incentives include all *except* which one of the following:**
    A. Hanging a copy of the Hippocratic Oath in a prominent position in the physician's office
    B. Informed consent, which involves information, understanding and noncoercion
    C. Disclosure of financial matters, including disclosure of conflicts of interest
    D. Regulations, such as reducing the frequency of financial incentive-related bonuses or increasing the time between financial feedback reports to physicians

16. **Promoting integrity in practice can be helped by:**
    A. Handing out simple, one-page discussions about how managed care works and how the physician's office is reimbursed
    B. Emphasizing that the doctor's first loyalty is to the patient, but that he/she must still live within the rules
    C. Readily and actively help the patient to use any and all appeal processes whenever a patient's personal medical interest is at risk
    D. All of the above

17. **Which of the following statements is correct?**
    A. To intrude into a person's privacy, the state must show a compelling interest
    B. It is illegal for any private company to obtain confidential information about anyone
    C. Federal protection of electronic information is detailed and strict
    D. No states have, as yet, passed laws to limit or eliminate gag rules that prohibit physicians from discussing diagnostic, therapeutic or consultative options that are not covered by the patient's managed care organization

18. **When a doctor treats a patient in a managed care context, he/she can protect the patient's privacy best by:**
   A. Keeping no notes whatsoever
   B. Keeping secret any information that a patient reveals or requests be kept secret that does not bear directly on clinically significant issues
   C. Informing the patient beforehand that anything the physician is told will go into the record
   D. Avoid asking patients any personal questions, such as any stress they may be experiencing, even if it might be important to an understanding of their medical condition

19. **Which of the following statements is correct?**
   A. A Pennsylvania patient's employer was found liable for inappropriately using HIV prescription information (obtained from a pharmacy benefit manager) against the patient
   B. Physicians should always tell their patients that the drug they are prescribing, while perfectly effective, is not the best drug for their condition but is the one permitted in the formulary by the plan, when such is the case
   C. Only 40 percent of all prescriptions written are filled, and compliance falls as dosing frequency diminishes
   D. All of the above

20. **According to the author, the principle of beneficence (doing good for the patient) under managed care:**
   A. Continues to take precedence over all other ethical principles and remains a disease-centered effort rather than becoming more person- and population-centered
   B. Will probably come to look a lot more like self-help, as the principle of autonomy assumes greater prominence
   C. Is directly at odds with any effort to provide cost-effective treatments
   D. Encourages the rising use of what is known as "futile treatment"

21. Which of the following statements is correct?
   A. The most common cause of medication error is the use of computer software, rather than total reliance on old-fashioned handwritten prescriptions
   B. About 9 percent of prescriptions are effectively queried by pharmacists
   C. Pharmacists should avoid all educational efforts to inform patients about medications, since they are not physicians
   D. The challenge to find ways to keep patient identification related to medication more confidential should not be a concern for pharmacists

22. The three ethical questions posed by the author relating to the role of house physicians include which of the following:
   A. Should the house physician–patient relationship carry the same obligations as any other physician–patient relationship?
   B. Should the house physician owe first loyalty to patient, attending physician, or managed care payer?
   C. Should the attending physician be compensated for the house physician's efforts?
   D. All of the above

23. Marginal treatments:
   A. Are defined as therapies, medications or devices that offer minimal potential benefit and effectiveness to a particular patient, given his/her medical condition
   B. Tend to be overutilized in managed care settings
   C. Are treatments to which every patient has a right
   D. Are defined as treatments that will be neither medically effective nor personally beneficial for any particular patient

24. Which of the following statements is correct?
   A. At least two Circuit Courts have suggested that there is a constitutionally protected right to die
   B. The Supreme Court has ruled that all Americans have an absolute right to medical treatment

   C. There is no ruling that requires HMOs and hospitals, among others, to ask whether patients have advance directives

   D. All of the above

25. **Inasmuch as physician-assisted suicide is not medically acceptable and not a constitutional right, physicians should:**

   A. Never withhold life-support systems, even when requested to do so in advance directives

   B. Always offer both marginal and futile treatments, and when these are not covered by any particular managed care plan, fight to have them allowed

   C. Become more skilled at pain control and communicate better with patients about their fears, such as fears of suffocating, becoming a burden or suffering

   D. Covertly engage in helping patients commit suicide if that fulfills their own personal ethic

26. **With regard to advance directives:**

   A. Physicians are much better than family members at guessing what a patient's real preference may be for life-sustaining treatment

   B. In most cases, hospital clinicians will be intimately familiar with patients' advance directives

   C. The real danger of advance directives in managed care is that they may be used to limit needed, useful, but expensive treatment under the guise of ethics

   D. They are routinely ignored anyway and hence serve no purpose

27. **To ensure the successful and ethical use of advance directives, they must be:**

   A. Discussed with both the patient and his/her proxy, if possible, together, in the same office visit, and become part of the patient's annual history and physical health assessment

   B. Interpreted in light of a patient's current decision-making capacity, and if that is impaired, his/her potential for recovering that capacity

C. A major part of a managed care organization's community educational effort, *focused on understanding patient values*

D. All of the above

28. **Practical rules for reducing the risk of malpractice suits in managed care practice include all *except* which of the following:**

A. Never change a patient's medical record, except by lining through an entry, initialing it and dating it

B. Never call patients when they miss appointments

C. Minimize all communications with patients so one cannot possibly be misunderstood

D. Recognize that ethical problems and legal problems have nothing to do with each other

29. **Which of the following is not one of the ways suggested by the author to enhance respect between doctor and patient?**

A. Orient patients to the process of the visit when they first come in

B. Try not to make patients feel rushed or ignored

C. Laugh more at patients, even at their own expense

D. Give more information about lifestyle and the psychosocial aspects of care

30. **Which of the following types of incentives may be considered ethical?**

A. Negative incentives that simply save the employer or the HMO money while putting the doctor and patient in adversarial positions

B. Financial conflicts of interest that adversely affect clinical judgment

C. Negative incentives to provide care that utilize general considerations of cost, benefit and effectiveness data

D. Threats of deselection (termination of the physician's employment) for revealing treatment options or financial issues that the profit-oriented HMO does not want to have discussed with patients

31. In order to promote the principle of fairness to all involved in managed care, a physician can:
A. Acknowledge that the conflict between fidelity to an individual patient and the greatest good for the greatest number of patients is a central part of the managed care philosophy
B. Be sure patients are encouraged and supported in their efforts to appeal whenever treatment is unfairly denied
C. Become expert on at least one preventive topic as a way to prevent illness, improve the ability to provide for others, and extend the available capitated resources
D. All of the above

32. Which of the following statements is correct?
A. So far, courts have generally ruled in favor of managed care plans when sued by patients, even if treatment limitations appeared unclear or decidedly unfair
B. One solid approach to integrating the principle of fairness with that of autonomy is to be as unscientific as possible in one's approach to medical practice
C. The safest ethical (and legal) position for the physician working in a managed care setting is to be an individual patient advocate first and foremost
D. All of the above

33. The Picker Institute's "patient-centered questions" survey showed that patients:
A. Who are younger and/or male tend to be more satisfied with physicians and with hospital care than older and/or female patients
B. Value communication of information about health or medical treatment actually more than physicians do

C. Are much more concerned with the hotel-like services hospitals offer than with the quality of medical/physician care

D. Prefer not to have any involvement in their care by friends or family members

34. **Which of the following issues are cited in the JCAHO's 1998 accreditation standards which emphasize patient rights and require institutions to implement "an ethics process to deal with ethical issues"?**
A. Forgoing life-sustaining treatment
B. Resolving disagreements in care decisions
C. Participating in clinical trials
D. All of the above

35. **The most common reasons physicians currently ask for ethics services include all except which of the following?**
A. Evaluating a patient's decision-making capacity
B. Formulating, interpreting, and implementing advance directives, as well as the matter of withdrawing or withholding treatment
C. Disagreements with the managed care organization with regard to their salaries or other financial arrangements
D. Resolving disagreements among health care professionals, patients and families

36. **In the inpatient setting, newer ethical issues arising from the managed care context focus on:**
A. Billing, coding and referring problems
B. Questions about marginal care and who should pay for it
C. Appealing financial constraints on a patient's treatment
D. All of the above

INDEX

A

Access to treatment
Medicare patients, 53
suicide and, 115
uninsured people, 34, 46, 97, 140, 142
Accountability, 15–23
arguments against, 22–23
arguments for, 21–22
autonomy and, 17–18
patient commitment, 16–17
physician commitment, 17
Acupuncture, 90
Advance directives in managed care, 12, 45,
120–123
altruistic motivation, 121–122
danger of, 122–123
description, 120–121
financial motivation, 122–123
living wills, 12, 120
Advertising by physicians, 81
Advocacy. *See* Patient advocacy by physicians
African-Americans, 48–50
advance directives and, 121
Alcohol abuse, 22
Alternative medicine, ethical questions
concerning, 77, 89–92
contextual factors, 91
patient preferences, 90–91
quality-of-life factors, 92
safety, 89
American Indians. *See* Native Americans
American Medical Association (AMA)
Code of Ethics, 152
Council on Ethical and Judicial Affairs, 152
American Medical News, 31, 56, 91, 176
Annals of Internal Medicine, 92
Annas, George, 110
Anti-disparagement clauses, 10, 64
Appeal process, physician use of, 59, 171
Asian-Americans, 48–49, 51
advance directives and, 121

B

Barnett v. Kaiser Foundation Health Plan, Inc., 180
Behavior, changing, 174
Beneficence in a managed care context, 73–80
alternative medicine and, 90
case example, 73, 78
futile treatment, 75–76
future possibilities, 78–80
gatekeeping, 76–77
marginal treatment, 77
process rather than outcome, 75
Billing, 155–156
Blue Cross/Blue Shield use of Milliman and
Robertson guidelines, 29
Bonuses, physician, 151–152
Burzynski, Stanislaw, 89

C

California, leader in managed care legislation,
86–87
Capitation, 11, 151
end-of-life care and, 12
informed consent and. *See* Informed consent and capitation
Medicare patients, 52
Case-based education, 192
Cassel, Christine, 118
Celebrity factor in organ allocation, 185
"Churning," 155
CIGNA use of Milliman and Robertson
guidelines, 29
Clinical Medical Ethics, 126
Clinical service, hospital ethics programs, 192
CME, 195–207

A (second column)

Assisted suicide. *See* Suicide and managed care
Attorney, patient, 29, 161. *See also* Legal
considerations and ethics
Autonomy
of patients. *See* Patient autonomy
of physicians, 8